A

Seed

of Hope

A Fertility Devotional

Revised Edition

Evangeline Brown Colbert

A Seed of Hope---God's Promises of Fertility
Published by Seed of Faith Ministries | iHope Publishing
Copyright © 2011 Evangeline Colbert; Revised Edition © 2017

ISBN: 978-0-9858303-4-2

Contents

DISCLAIMER:

The content published in this book is solely for informational purposes. Nothing contained in this book or any additional linked sources is intended to constitute legal, health, or other professional advice. You should consult with an appropriate professional for specific advice tailored to your situation. Evangeline Colbert is not a medical professional and does not intend, by anything she says in this book, to be dispensing medical/psychological advice to the reader.

You should consult a physician before changing you medication or discontinuing any prescribed treatment. Any health advice adopted from this book by the reader is done at his or her own risk. If additional legal advice, or mental/physical health advice is needed, seek the advice of your legal/health professional.

Neither the author of this book nor the publisher has any liability whatsoever in regard to loss, damage, or injury suffered directly or indirectly as a result of the information contained in this book.

Readers' Praise for
A Seed of Hope

I love this book!! It is helping me get through this tough time. There are a lot words of encouragement and most importantly God's word and promise!!! I would recommend this to anyone going through infertility. If I could I would hand them out. That's how much I love this book.
~Kristin H.

I am a woman who is experiencing infertility. I have been through years of trying, and this has caused me to end up with depression and no hope. I found this book while I was searching for Christian infertility sites. Since I have purchased this book, my whole outlook on my current situation has changed! I am now a woman full of hope who is believing that God is working on a miracle in my life. This book has spoken God's word to me, and now I am living a hopeful life, speaking His word in my daily walk with Him. If you or anyone that you know is going through the pain of infertility, I highly recommend this book! It is my nightly encouragement!
~Angie

Even though it is written for those with infertility issues, the Scriptures speak to life issues such as trusting the Lord to supply all that we need... Evangeline's encouragement is from the place she has been and lets us know we also can trust God for our deliverance, no matter what the situation looks like. I love her book!
~Linda C.

Foreword
By Elisha Kearns

I am not sure if you are new to infertility or if you have been traveling this journey for months or even years, but I think we can all agree no matter the time spent on this unexpected path to parenthood that it is tough. *Really tough.* When I began walking this bumpy road filled with sharp turns and potholes, I wasn't prepared. Were you?

I thought infertility was simply the inability to conceive after one year of actively trying. And rightfully so, because isn't that the definition? But ask me now, nearly six years after leaving my doctor's office numb and confused, then going through several failed treatment cycles and a miscarriage, and I will quickly tell you that the definition Google search gave me years ago is not even close to being accurate, and maybe you feel the same. Infertility, when you break it down, is *so much more* than just the inability to conceive.

I have learned it is also a series of losses that you are forced to grieve month after month. It's almost like a grave that keeps following you around as it grabs your hope and buries more and more of your dreams with each failed cycle. It's a fierce battle between your faith and your circumstances. A battle you must fight to win every day. And a battle that is exhausting. But sweet friend, while I have learned so much about infertility through my experiences, I have also learned what it is not. And it is not going to win.

In 2012 after my last failed treatment cycle using In Vitro-Fertilization (IVF), I found myself falling further into a sea of despair thinking God had forgotten me. I couldn't figure out what I had done to deserve this form of punishment and this type of shame. Every day, I felt as though I was trying to scoop the water out of my sinking ship with a small Dixie cup, only to keep watching the water come pouring back in.

It wasn't until during one of my late night internet searches in which I was looking for something, anything that could give me relief from the intense pain my heart and soul was experiencing that I found her; I found Evangeline and her book, *A Seed of Hope: God's Promises for Fertility*. And friend, once it was in my hands just a few short days later, I couldn't put it down. Each entry was a breath of spiritual fresh air as her words brought life to the parts of me that were dry and wounded.

I found her personal struggle and unwavering faith in God to be the powerful inspiration I needed in my time of weakness. Her daily dose of encouragement helped me shake off the lies of the enemy so that I could stand firm and live my day faithfully with a hope-filled focus. A focus that has continued to enable me to believe in the Truth that victory over childlessness, no matter the diagnosis or cause, can be mine— and even yours.

It is my prayer and strong belief that as you dedicate each day to reading this 60-day devotional, as well as put to practice the undeniable tool of speaking God's word over your situation as Evangeline teaches you to do, that you will begin to feel your hope supernaturally rise to a new level. You will begin to see yourself *with* the victory, rather than without. I also believe that you will begin to feel stronger in your faith, as well as empowered to know that while infertility is what it is— heartbreaking...dream shattering...soul crushing and faith breaking...you will also begin to know deep down within your spirit what it is not. You will know that because of the power of Jesus, it is not going to win.

So grab a pen, a cute journal and marinate yourself with the Spirit-filled words of this book. Let it be a tool that helps you no longer see your situation through your eyes, but rather through His. You are a victor through Him, and victory over sickness and disease can be yours.

Thank you, Evangeline, for pouring out your heart and spreading God's Truth to a community of men and women struggling to conceive. Your dedication to the Lord years ago saved me from turning away from my faith. My hope and prayer today is that through your revised edition, it will continue to help save others who are like I once was— trying to scoop water out of their boat with a small Dixie cup.

May God bless each of you reading these words with the deepest desires of your heart.

Elisha Kearns
Author of the faith-based nationally known blog, Waiting for Baby Bird

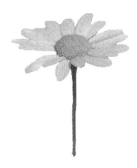

For Jesus Christ, the
Son of God, does not
waver between "Yes"
and "No." He is the
one whom Silas,
Timothy, and I
preached to you, and
as God's ultimate
"Yes," He always
does what He says."

2 Corinthians 1:19 NLT

Introduction

The pain of infertility hurts worse than the pain of delivering a baby. I have experienced both sources of pain. The intense pain of infertility can last for many months or even years and hurts at depths within your soul that can eventually challenge your sense of completeness as a woman. Labor and delivery of a baby typically cause intense pain only within your body and usually lasts less than 24 hours. My experience with both sources of pain has given me a platform from which I can offer hope for victory to women who are struggling with infertility.

I want to share with you, and those that you know and love who may be in the struggle of overcoming childlessness, that through faith in Jesus and speaking the Word of God, I am a three-time victor in that struggle. I want to make it clear to you that *there is hope!* The Word of God is the source of hope in my life and was the source of my victory over infertility.

For my husband and me, infertility began as a process of suffering repeated disappointment month after month. Because I had always experienced heavy and painful menstrual periods since my teens, we decided to seek medical advice. Ultrasound examinations and blood tests were ordered and eventually laparoscopic surgery was suggested. When we first heard the doctor's report of the test results, we were not quite sure what to do or how to handle what he told us. He predicted a negative outcome—that we may never have children. Waves of disbelief, fear, and sadness came quickly to my mind. We sat in his office in shock, having never anticipated his report. I was 27 years old and had never had a gynecologist give me any indication this prognosis was a possibility.

But God was faithful. He began to take me through a process that would later produce a different outcome. The process was one of learning how to trust Him more, to use His Word as a tool, and to persevere to victory. Contrary to the doctor's prediction, I became pregnant and we now have three beautiful children who love God and are blessings to us and to their community.

Be encouraged! This book is for you, so you will see you no longer need to remain in bondage to infertility or childlessness. My hope is that by reading these devotions daily, they will serve to increase your awareness of the importance of speaking and believing the Word of God over *any* situation in your life. God made it possible for you to use His Word to make your affirmation of faith in Him and affect change in your circumstances. The intent of this book is to always point you to Jesus Christ and the wonderful promises He made to you in His Word so you can increase your hope and see His promises of children manifested in your life.

Use this book and God's Truth contained in it to share in the victory that Jesus has already won on your behalf when He gave His life for you. Use it as a resource as you study your Bible. Do "treasure hunts" in the Bible to find scriptures that hold God's special promises for you. It will build your confidence in the victory that Jesus secured for you because God's Word *can* change your present circumstances.

As you begin and continue to speak the promises of God that relate to your health and fertility, remember that the confession is not a magic wand. **You are not confessing His Word to** *get* **the promised blessing. You are confessing His promises because you are in Christ and therefore they are** *already* **yours.**

Believe **you have already been blessed with what He promised and provided through Jesus' finished work on the cross (Mark 11:24; Ephesians 1:3).**

I pray that this book will move you to action; allow the Holy Spirit to help you use your faith to produce action that corresponds to having a greater level of confidence in Jesus. This book is based on God's principle of what I call "spoken faith." In other words, speaking the Word of God while believing the Word of God and trusting in His love for you (Romans 10:9,10). Included are suggested action points called "Confidence in Action". Use them as a means to start taking additional steps of faith that indicate you believe you are an overcomer of infertility.

No matter what, continue to point your faith towards the Father's love for you and receive His grace. That was His reason for sending Jesus---to demonstrate His love and put you in a position to receive everything good in life, including children. As you increasingly realize and accept how much God loves you, and as you take the time to tap into His strength that is found in His Word, your confidence in Jesus will soar!

"Therefore do not cast away your confidence, which has great reward. For you have need of endurance, so that after you have done the will of God, you may receive the promise." ~ Hebrews 10:35, 36

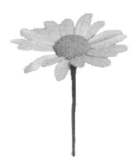

"There has not failed
one word of all His
good promise..."
    1 Kings 8:56

How to Use This Book

This revised version of A Seed of Hope *incorporates some changes to the content so that it's more interactive and, I hope, beneficial. Now you'll find questions at the end of each daily reading so that you can "**Dig Deeper**". Some of them may be a bit challenging but work through them— doing so will build your faith. These questions can also be used for support group meetings as prompts to additional discussion.*

Read an entry daily, being sure to pay attention to and meditate on each opening scripture. Each devotion will end with three sections:

> **Speak the Word**—*Say this section out loud.* It is usually based on the opening scripture. God's Word is alive and brings light to our lives (Psalm 119:130). It builds our faith as we hear it more and more, especially when we hear it from our own mouth (Romans 10:17).

> **More Encouragement**—Additional scriptures are provided so that you can read and study to reinforce what you've read in the devotion.

> **Dig Deeper**—This will be a question for you to consider as you anticipate God's promises of fertility bringing His truth into manifestation.

Each day's devotion will have some scripture references embedded in the text. Enjoy some time with the Lord by looking them up in your bible and then allow them to bless your mind, your spirit, and of course, your body!

Confidence in Action

Wherever you see these "Confidence in Action" pages, they contain suggestions for you to take actions of faith that correspond with your asking and believing God for deliverance from infertility. Your actions will reflect that you believe you receive what you've asked for, according to His Word. Demonstrate your confidence in the promises of God!

For further study:

Mark 11:23, 24 and 1 John 5:14, 15

These pages will also provide a "Reflections" section where you can write your thoughts, prayers and plans. Record the encouragement, revelations, and new ideas God gives you as you meditate on His Word.

A number of scriptures that are particularly applicable to fertility are included in the **Appendix** for you to use for daily meditation on the ability of God to make you fruitful.

A Personal Note to You

I first began to write this book in 2004, in the form of a booklet, as a way to share the precious nuggets of God's Word about overcoming infertility. My goal was two-fold:

1) To promote the truth that NOTHING is too hard for God, and

2) To help women understand that God's healing hand **still** moves on their behalf, no matter what the doctor's report may be.

For me, obtaining peace of mind and standing in victory over infertility were each accomplished because of the Word of God. I poured over the scriptures, finding those that related to infertility, faith, and being a mother. I read them regularly to remind myself of God's love for me and of His willingness to change my circumstances.

In 2009, I knew that God was prompting me to expand the booklet to give an even wider view of how He wants women to use His Word when they are dealing with infertility (and anything else in life). This book should enable you to take **"daily doses" of encouragement** from those same scriptures I used many years ago.

I hope that you will begin seeing more of God's character in His promises—always loving, always willing, and always being faithful to say "Yes" to them. Trust Him as a Promise keeper.

My prayer is that as you read this book you will be greatly encouraged, recognizing that victory starts in your mind and is enforced by your mouth speaking the Word of God. I pray that you also will stand as an overcomer, prevailing over infertility through faith in God's love for you and in the power of His Word, ultimately birthing and raising godly sons and daughters.

Grace and Peace,
Evangeline

"Is any thing too hard for the LORD?" Genesis 18:14

Exercising Your Faith

*"He did not waver at the promise of God through unbelief,
but was strengthened in faith, giving glory to God..."*

~ Romans 4:20 ~

Does your faith need some building up in order to believe God for conquering infertility? Consider the life of Abraham. When he was 100 and his wife, Sarah, was 90, they were still childless. They had to continue to believe God would do what He promised them almost 25 years earlier... to make Abraham the father of many nations through a child from Sarah's body.

Abraham strengthened his faith in that promise by giving God praise (Romans 4:19-21). He praised God as a means to remind himself of what God promised and what He was capable of. You should do the same, especially at those times when you think, "I'll never get pregnant", "What's wrong with me?" or, "Maybe I'm not supposed to have any children." That's when you have to remind yourself and convince yourself that God is able to do anything and that nothing, not even infertility, is impossible with Him on your side.

You may wonder if God really is on your side. Well, if you've asked Jesus to be your Savior, God is and will always be on your side. You are in covenant with Him and He will *always* honor that. If you have not asked Jesus to be your Savior, would you stop and do that now by praying this simple prayer out loud?

> *Dear God in heaven, I ask you to forgive me of the wrong things I've done. I believe that you love me as I am and that Jesus died and rose from the dead for my benefit. I ask Jesus to come into my heart and be Lord over my life. I want everything you have for my life. Thank you in Jesus' name, Amen.*

If you prayed that prayer... Congratulations! You're now and forever a child of God and a recipient of His abundant grace and love. You can partake of every good and every perfect gift God already had planned for you. His plan for you is wonderful, filled with blessing without measure!

Now, back to the story of Abraham---Abraham knew that continually reminding himself of who God was and what He had promised to him was the way to avoid doubt and unbelief. He was able to "keep the faith" no matter what his current circumstances were. He's a great example of having faith that doesn't waver. He stayed focused on the promise, not on the problem of infertility. He believed God and praised his way out of his circumstance.

It's because of Jesus that you can rest assured that the God of the entire universe is on your side. That's a good reason to praise Him. There's no need to fear what the future holds. If God is for you, then who can successfully be against you (Romans 8:31)? That's *another* good reason to praise Him! Continue to think about all the ways God has previously come through for you. Continue to think about all the reasons that you can count on Him.

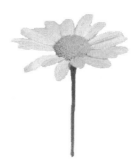

Speak the Word: I praise and thank God for all He's done and all that He promised me. I am fully persuaded that what Jesus has promised, He is also able *and* willing to perform.

More Encouragement: Hebrews 11:1-2, 8-11; Mark 1:41

Dig Deeper: In what ways have you struggled with unbelief about any of God's promises of fertility? How have you addressed this?

You Have His Word

*"Blessed be the Lord, that has given rest to his people
Israel, according to all that he promised. Not one word has
failed of all His good promise..."*
~1 Kings 8:56 (AMP) ~

D o you have "trust issues"? We as women tend to
have many "issues" and trust is a big one. It's so
much easier to trust someone who has never lied
nor failed to do what they've promised than it is to trust
someone who never does what they say they'll do. Well,
there's good news. Nothing that God has spoken has ever
failed. None of His promises have ever failed. Not even
one! Isn't it wonderful to know that God never has and
never will lie to you? The Bible assures us of that in
Hebrews 6:18, Titus 1:2, and Numbers 23:19. You can
place your trust and confidence in Him—He will *always*
come through on what He has promised.

But what if He doesn't do it in your timing? Are you patient
enough to wait for His promise to be manifested? Will you
rest in Him and not be anxious? Can you endure and hold
on to the promise of a child even when you continue to
have your menstrual cycle month after month after month?
It may feel like the hardest thing you've ever had to endure,
but the good thing is if you've accepted Jesus as Savior,
His Spirit lives in you. His Spirit leads you and comforts
you so that each day is easier to get through because you
acknowledge that He's on your side. Jesus loves you so
much. He is always there to strengthen you and to help you

to hold on to your joy. He's there when friends have given up on believing for you. He's even there when family members say, "Are you ever going to have any children? You're not getting any younger you know!"

Despite what you hear from others, *choose* to continue to believe in the power of God's Word and to view it as His collection of personal promises to you. Search His Word and find yourself in it; find His promises that speak directly to you so when you see them they make you say, "That's me!" Then trust Him and *speak* that Word because He has said to put His Word in your mouth and your heart (Romans 10:8).

God is trustworthy. His promises are sure. None of them will fail!

Speak the Word: I believe in the power of God's Word. I trust that what God has said is sure to bring transformation to my life.

More Encouragement: Isaiah 40:5; Isaiah 55:11; Joshua 23:14

Dig Deeper: God's character is a model of trustworthiness. What challenges you most about resting in His love for you?

Speaking the Word

"For You have exalted above all else Your name and Your word and You have magnified Your word above all Your name!"
~ *Psalm 138:2 (AMP)* ~

In the beginning was the Word...
God created this planet and the entire universe by *speaking* it into existence. His words contain power! As believers in Jesus Christ, and therefore as children of God, we can, like earthly children, imitate our heavenly Father by saying what He says.

We have the honor and privilege to use what God has said to create a life that falls in line with His plan for us---an abundant, overflowing life (Romans 10:8; John 10:10). *That abundance includes having children* and raising them to know that God loves them immensely and wants them to enjoy an abundant life (Psalm 102:18, 28).

We can activate that abundant life and change our current circumstances by believing and declaring God's Word. He gave us His Word to empower us so that we don't have to live in bondage to infertility any longer! Over and over again, God shows us in the Bible that it is important to speak His Word because it is powerful in shaping our lives.

God said that His Word would go forth and return to Him with results that please him (Isaiah 55:11). The method by which His Word returns to Him is through us speaking it out loud in faith. Everyone knows that God's name is holy and should be respected and honored. But did you know that He has exalted His Word even above His name (Psalm 138:2)? That means we should believe His Word, trust it, and value it as something precious! It also means we can act on it with **confidence**.

Speak God's Word and be encouraged that it is working and *will* work on your behalf. Believe it and continually speak it in faith (2 Corinthians 4:13). Speak the Word because it is the foundation for God's language of faith.

It's important to continually make scriptural affirmations. If you're wondering why repeatedly speaking the Word is so powerful, it's because when we speak the Word, we're in agreement with God! We're actually saying what He has already said about us. In the Amplified Bible version of Proverbs 22:17,18, we're instructed to "Listen (consent and submit) to the words of the wise, and apply your mind to knowledge; for it will be pleasant if you keep them in your mind [believing them]; your lips will be [accustomed] to confessing them."

David, a man who so openly loved and trusted God, knew the power of speaking the Word. He said in Psalm 17:4, "...By the word of Your lips, I have kept away from the paths of the destroyer." Similarly, we must speak the Word of God to keep us off of Satan's paths that are lined with his burdens and devices of deception.

Most importantly, speaking the Word helps us to keep our eyes and mind on Jesus' love for us, enabling us to receive the victory over infertility.

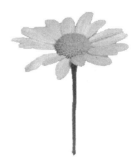

Speak the Word: I speak the Word of God because it is alive and powerful, and it keeps me from the destroyer's path of infertility.

More Encouragement: John 15:5; Romans 4:17; 2Corinthians 1:20

Dig Deeper: What are you thoughts about the power of God's Word and the effect it can have on your fertility? How can speaking His Word be incorporated into your daily lifestyle?

God's Circle of Blessing

"I will bless you richly. I will multiply your descendants…"
~ Genesis 22:17 ~

The Living Bible Translation of Psalm 25:13 says, "He shall live within God's circle of blessing, and his children shall inherit the earth."

To whom is this passage referring? The previous verse tells us…the person who reverences God.

Living in God's circle of blessing enables us to enjoy the best in life even when circumstances around us tell, and sometimes yell, otherwise. Isaac, Abraham's son, was a great example of living in the circle of blessing. The Bible's account in Genesis 26:1-13 tells how there was a famine in the country where Isaac lived and he wondered if he should leave like so many others and go to Egypt where there was no famine. God told him to stay and that He would be with Isaac in his obedience. God promised him increase in all areas of life, including children.

So in the midst of his country's famine, despair, lack, and death, Isaac was blessed with extreme abundance because he stayed where God wanted him—in His circle of blessing. Infertility is like a famine—extreme hunger and despair—except it's for a child. Just as Isaac experienced great bounty in the midst of famine, so can you, when you choose to remain in God's circle of blessing even as your circumstances scream "famine."

You can live in God's circle of blessing by keeping the ears of your heart open to His Word. Hear Him as He speaks to you through it. Receive the Word by faith, as personal promises from God to you. Receive His wonderful blessings by saying "thank you" to Him for the promises you find in his Word for your child. Repeatedly speak His Word, His Truth, over your life. When we speak the Word, we're in agreement with God. Receive His blessings by living in His Word and resting in His grace.

No matter what the doctor's reports say, you don't have to be *stuck* in the famine of infertility. Declare that you live in God's circle of blessing because famine can't exist there. Jesus is God of abundant joy! Nothing is too hard for Him to change; therefore He can change your circumstance of infertility. His Truth, His Word, can bring extreme abundance in its most wonderful form—the blessing of a child.

Speak the Word: I choose to stay in God's circle of blessing. He is my source of everything good.

More Encouragement: Galatians 3:14; Hebrews 6:14

Dig Deeper: What is a way you can rest in God's grace, knowing that He encircles you with blessings and His love?

Is Anything Too Hard for the Lord?

"But Jesus looked at them and said to them, "With men this is impossible, but with God all things are possible."
~ *Matthew 19:26* ~

In Genesis 18:14, God asks Abraham, "Is anything too hard for the Lord?"

In other words, He asked, "Is there anything that is so difficult, so big, so arduous, that I can't do it?" Do you think your state of infertility is beyond God's power? Is it really beyond His reach?

God is bigger than any problem that we face. The Bible declares there is nothing that exists without Him— everything started in Him, finds purpose in Him and is held together by Him. When you identify with the truth spoken by Jesus, you are able to use His truth to overcome any lie the devil whispers to you. Jesus wants us to be encouraged by the truth that He is able to change and improve *any* situation.

Abraham took hold of what God said, believed it as truth and lived in its fullness. He and Sarah were delivered from barrenness at the ages of 100 and 90, respectively— infertility was not too hard for God. And it *still* isn't! Believe that God wants wholeness in your life—that means in your body, your mind, your spirit, your finances, and your relationships.

Consider your life God's work zone and allow Him to start fresh and fabricate the "blueprint of hope" He has given to you for becoming a mom.

Others may consider infertility a permanent condition and not have confidence in God's love and ability. But rest assured, NOTHING IS TOO DIFFICULT FOR GOD!

Speak the Word: My God is GREAT and He loves me! No problem, condition, or circumstance in my life is too big or too difficult for God to change.

More Encouragement: Jeremiah 32:17, 27; Philippians 2:9-11,13

Dig Deeper: Be honest with yourself. On a scale of 1-10, how confident are you that God loves you? What can help you tap into His " blueprint of hope" for *your* life?

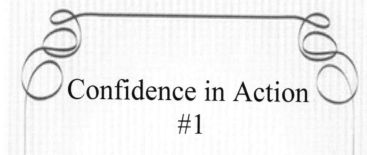

Confidence in Action
#1

Speak God's Word *daily*. Find scriptures that are directly related to overcoming infertility and speak them out loud. Decide that because you are made in God's image you will do as God does...declaring the desired end results from the beginning of a matter (Isaiah 46:9, 10). Nothing is too hard for Him so speak His Word into any dark circumstances so that LIFE and LIGHT can be brought into them (Job 22:28).

To get you started, a selection of scriptures is included in the Appendix.

Reflections

_____

_____

_____

_____

_____

_____

_____

_____

_____

_____

_____

_____

_____

_____

_____

_____

_____

_____

_____

None Barren

*"You shall be blessed above all people; there shall not be
male or female barren among you."*
~ Deuteronomy 7:14 (AMP) ~

G od said He wants men and women to be fruitful and
multiply (Genesis 1:28). His desire is for humanity
to produce godly, prosperous families. He loves us
so much and He wants to bless us abundantly. One of His
many blessings includes having children.

Many times, when childlessness / infertility ("barrenness"
as it is called in the Bible) strikes a husband and wife, the
couple's focus tends to only be on their inability to
reproduce. Proverbs 23:7 declares that what a person
continually thinks about is what he/she becomes. This
means what we put our attention to, or what we focus on
the most will expand in our lives. What you think about
over and over and over again is what will eventually
manifest in your life. This suggests that focusing on your
present inability to conceive will not change it but may
prolong it.

That's why it's imperative that you focus on God and not
on the problem of infertility. But what if your husband
doesn't share the hope you have? Do you discount him,
abandon him, ignore him or do you choose to be God's
example to him? Even if your husband's unbelief is an
issue for you, it's important for you to continue to stand on

God's Word and to engage other believers to stand with you.

In the Bible's account of Abraham and Sarah, Abraham didn't focus on his own impotence and say, "It's hopeless. This hundred year old body could never father a child." Nor was he discouraged by Sarah's decades of infertility and completely give up on the hope of having a child with her. He focused on God's promise to him, confident that God would make good on what He said.

Think and meditate with confidence on His promise in Deuteronomy 7:14. Have confidence in God's *unconditional* love for you. Barrenness is not what God desires for His children. Have confidence that He wants you to be fruitful.

Speak the Word: God loves me unconditionally. I focus on His love for me. I am blessed and enjoy living in the favor of God. I am fruitful in my body.

More Encouragement: Deuteronomy 7:12-15

Dig Deeper: What steps can you take so that you're focused on God's promises of fertility and not on your problems?

Hope in God

"Hope in God and wait expectantly for Him. For I will yet praise Him who is the health of my countenance and my God." ~ Psalms 42:11 (AMP) ~

The Word tells us that every good gift, and every perfect gift flows to us from our Heavenly Father (James 1:17). That includes having children! It's a good reason to keep your hope in God. Months or years of waiting to become pregnant are painful. It's important to guard against falling into a trap where painful thoughts lead to depression.

We should continue to praise God even through our troubles. The pressure of trouble in our lives produces patience when we *choose* to maintain our joy, a positive attitude, and endure. As we patiently endure, we build and continue in hope. Maintaining hope produces a habit of *joyful* expectation. Hope in God never disappoints. Hope is one of the three things that 1 Corinthians 13:13 tells us will always remain as a resource that allows us to tap into God's grace. We are to *always* have hope—the joyful and confident expectation of God coming through for us!

One of the best ways to wait *expectantly* for God and to maintain your hope in Him is to praise Him. Praising God brings and keeps your soul (your mind, will, and emotions) out of depression. Praise is a source of strength. It is an exercise that changes your countenance and outlook on life. Praise is simply verbally telling God that you admire Him,

34

value Him, and that you are grateful for Him being in your life and thankful for all He's done. Praise is enthusiastically telling God that He is The Greatest and without Him you would be nothing. Thank Him for the gifts of healing, prosperity, and salvation that all come to you through His Son, Jesus. Praise is acknowledging and saying that *all* your blessings flow from Him and that He has a purpose for your life.

Make the choice to use praise to encourage yourself and elevate your level of hope. Even as you wait for the manifestation of your desire for a child, *expect* God to come through on His promises. His blessing will continue to flow up to the limit of your expectation.

Allow Jesus to work without limits or boundaries in your life. *Expect* increase and be in a position to receive His good and His perfect gifts from Him. The Bible says that hope does not disappoint because "blessed is the man whose hope is the Lord (Jeremiah 17:7). *Expect* to receive the blessing of a child. *Expect great things from a GREAT GOD*!

Speak the Word: I maintain my hope in God. I will praise Him and grow in hope by the power of the Holy Spirit, regardless of my circumstances.

More Encouragement: Romans 15:13; Romans 5:3-5

Dig Deeper: What will you do to incorporate more praise and expectancy into your daily routine?

His Covenant of Love

"He will love you, bless you, and multiply you; He will also
bless the fruit of your body..."
~ Deuteronomy 7:13 ~

When dealing with infertility, it's important to know that God loves you immensely. Based on His great love for you and me, God established a blood covenant for us through the death of Jesus. A covenant is an agreement made by two parties, agreeing that all they possess in this life is available to the covenant partner upon demand. The covenant is until death and cannot be altered.

If you choose to accept His covenant and make Jesus your Lord and Savior, you are a partner in this never-ending covenant of love. God's covenant opens the way for you to receive His blessing, which you can receive because of His grace, through your faith in Jesus.

Accept and believe that God's love for you is unconditional. His love for you will not change. Isn't that good news? No matter what you've done wrong, He won't stop loving you. No matter how good you are He couldn't love you any more than He already does. His love for you is based on His love for Jesus, not on what you do or don't do.

Read scriptures about God's love for you (out loud, to yourself) as many times as it takes for His words to make their way from your head to your heart. By doing so, you position yourself to receive His love and effortlessly take hold of His blessings. You'll also develop a passion for the things of God and His words will become more real to you. You'll have more confidence in the concept that what He has said to you in the Bible is not only true; it is absolute. It is unchangeable. It is TRUTH.

Jesus has done and said it all so that you can take advantage of all that He is and of His *endless* supply of love!

Speak the Word: God accepts me as I am. He loves me, blesses me, and increases me. He blesses my children, which are the fruit of my body.

More Encouragement: John 17:23; Psalm 105:8; Romans 8:37-39

Dig Deeper: On a daily basis, how do you remind yourself of Jesus' endless supply of love toward you?

What Should I Do?

"If you need wisdom—if you want to know what God wants you to do—ask him, and he will gladly tell you. He will not resent your asking."
~ James 1:5 (NLT) ~

L ife can sometimes put us in situations where it's hard to know what to do or what our next step should be.

That's why it's always wise to pray and ask God for wisdom. Let Him know that you are submitting this situation of infertility to Him, because you have faith in what Jesus has done on your behalf on the cross and you're trusting that He will turn it around. God can give you specific instructions about what to do. He will give you your own special battle plan for victory (James 1:3-5).

The Word says in Proverbs 18:14 that your inner man, your spirit, needs to be strengthened in order for your body to be strengthened properly. You are strengthened in your inner man by communing with God, your spirit communicating with His Spirit. This includes, among other things, praying, reading and meditating on His Word, and singing songs about His love, grace and power.

There are of course, natural things that you can do that are effective alongside the spiritual things because your actions are actually a means of showing your active faith in God (James 2:26). See the "Confidence in Action" pages throughout this book. They contain ways of showing your confidence in how He has provided a way of escape from the condition of infertility.

Use this devotional as a tool; consider it as one of your weapons for battle. It serves as a resource for encouragement by offering multiple scriptures that specifically relate to infertility. Ultimately, knowing the right thing to do involves daily asking God for wisdom. His way will always be the best way. Let Him speak to you through His Word. Hebrews 4:12 states that God's Word is alive and powerful. It is able to change things. Let His Word be your change-agent in this situation of infertility. Your use of God's Word, by having faith in it and receiving wisdom through it, will have a major impact on turning infertility around.

Speak the Word: I ask God for wisdom and He gladly gives it to me.

More Encouragement: Proverbs 2:10; Proverbs 3:13

Dig Deeper: Wisdom is the principal thing. What do you need to ask God to give you wisdom about before proceeding to whatever is next?

Act "As If"

*"...God in whom he believed, Who gives life to the dead
and speaks of the nonexistent things that He has foretold
and promised as if they already existed."*
~ Romans 4:17 (AMP) ~

Having confidence in what God says helps you to take action and to have courage to live as if what His Word promises you already exists.

It actually does already exist in the spiritual realm and your faith in what He has said about being fertile is the means of accessing it so that it manifests in this natural realm.

You may have heard self-development teachers and speakers say if you want to be successful and prosperous, you need to "act as if" it's already so. Well, that way of thinking actually lines up with scripture and it's applicable to how you should deal with infertility. God does not desire nor expect you to live with or "accept the fate" of infertility. Romans 4:17 states that Abraham believed what God said to him about having a baby with his wife, Sarah, even though they were both over ninety years old. God is described as being the One who calls those things that be not as though they were.

In other words, God called forth and spoke about non-existent things "as if" they already existed. If that's God's way of doing things then, as a believer in Him, it should be our way of doing things too. After all, we are made in His image (Genesis 1:26).

Therefore, begin to act AND speak "as if" your body is fertile ground, ready and able to receive the seed that will produce life within you. Speak with confidence that God loves you unconditionally and is keeping His promise that He will bless the fruit of your body.

> *A Prayer of Faith*: God, I thank you that your love for me is unconditional. It does not depend on what I do or don't do. Your love for me is so deep and wonderful. Thank you that through your son Jesus, I receive every blessing you have for me. I choose to believe your Word and speak and act as if my body *is* fertile, as You intended it to be. I have confidence that You keep your promises.

Speak the Word: I call my body fertile because in His divine plan, God said He intended for none to be barren.

More Encouragement: Romans 4:17-21; Hebrews 11:3

Dig Deeper: What's the best way for you to "act as if" you expect your body to be fertile?

Confidence

*"Now thanks be to God, who always leads us in
triumph in Christ…"*
~ *2 Corinthians 2:14* ~

C onfidence. It means trusting in the abilities, strengths, integrity, or faithfulness of someone or some thing.

Typically, we willingly speak out boldly about people when we are confident in them. We are told in 1 John 5:14 that having confidence in God means that we believe that He hears us when we pray according to His Word and that He will grant what we ask. Part of your battle plan against infertility must include increasing your confidence in God's love for you.

Having confidence in others, even God, may sometimes be difficult. Have you ever had trouble letting someone else be in charge? I have. Have you ever wanted someone else to take control of a situation and allowed him or her to do so, only to snatch it right back because you didn't like how he or she was doing it?

Maybe that's what you're experiencing with God—not trusting Him enough to completely let go of your circumstances and allowing Him to be in control. If so, you've got to get over the fear of what will happen if you're not in control and instead, trust that His way is a better way. Develop a positive expectation of what will happen when *He's* in control.

That's what my husband and I experienced in our battle against infertility. As engineers, we both were good planners and detail-oriented. We had our lives planned out and thought we knew exactly when we'd start having children. We'd planned to wait until we had been married for 3-4 years, and of course we expected the pregnancy to happen within three months after we first started "trying".

On 6/2/86, I wrote in my journal: "Freeman and I are preparing to start pregnancy in July/August." Well, try as we may, our plan did not work. It didn't happen in July or August. Neither did it happen by the end of December. And so began the journey of going from doctor to doctor to see what was wrong with me and who could fix it. That journey did not last long before we decided we'd had enough. We clearly saw our need to develop confidence in God. We had to become better listeners to Him, through prayer and reading His Word, so we could follow *His* directions and find rest in *His* plan.

Speak the Word: I submit myself to God and His plan because I am confident that He always causes me to triumph in Christ Jesus.

More Encouragement: Hebrews 10:35, 36; 1 John 5:14,15

Dig Deeper: What are some practical ways that you build your confidence in the fact that Jesus' victory is also your victory?

Mama Knew Best

*"You will keep him in perfect peace, whose mind is stayed
on You, because he trusts in You.*
~ Isaiah 26:3 ~

I received a letter from my mother, dated January 21,
1987, encouraging me to not be anxious about the
doctor's reports, to trust in God, and to allow His peace
to overtake any worry. She wrote:

> *Dear Evangeline and Freeman,*
> *Regarding you wanting to have a child---that is very*
> *good. But don't be too concerned because it hasn't*
> *already happened. We cannot and should not try to*
> *rush God. And above all, we must be careful not to*
> *complain about it. Just pray about it, but don't*
> *worry about it. Leave it in the hands of the Lord.*
> *Try not to think about it. I do believe He is going to*
> *bless you with a child and you must believe that He*
> *will and leave the date to Him.*
>
> *I'm glad to hear you say you weren't going to go*
> *from doctor to doctor to find out why you haven't*
> *conceived. One of the verses which has really*
> *sustained me when I want something from God is*
> *found in Philippians 4:6-7 (RSV)---"Have no*
> *anxiety about anything, but in everything by prayer*
> *and supplication (requests) with thanksgiving let*
> *your requests be made known to God. And the*

peace of God which passes all understanding will keep your hearts and your minds in Christ Jesus."

By all means do not let the fact that your friends have children cause you to feel bad because you don't have any. You both have too much to be thankful for to complain...you're always in His care. He loves you both.

Love Always,

Mama

I hope her letter encourages you as much as it encouraged me. Be thankful. Refuse to worry. Enjoy living in His peace.

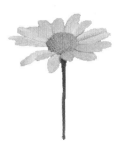

Speak the Word: I refuse to worry. I'm thankful that God's peace keeps my heart and mind.

More Encouragement: John 14:1; Philippians 2:13

Dig Deeper: What does peace of mind look and feel like for you?

The Power of Hope

"Uphold me according to Your word, that I may live; and do not let me be ashamed of my hope." ~ Psalm 119:116 ~

Hope is what forms the inner image of what you desire. You should always have an inner image of what you expect and desire in life. You should see in your mind's eye what you want to become your reality.

Hope allows your heart and mind to be captured by that inner image of what you desire. What do you fix your hope upon when it comes to getting pregnant? In your mind, do you *see* yourself pregnant? Do you *see* yourself enjoying a healthy pregnancy? Do you *see* yourself delivering a healthy baby? If you do, then you have hope!

Without hope, it's easy to feel completely alone when you're suffering through the disappointments and struggles of infertility. Even though your spouse is there to console you, you may still feel like this burden is only on you. That it's your fault no baby has been conceived. That it's your fault the grandparents wannabes have a hard time being around you without asking, "Why don't we have any grandchildren yet?" You may even sometimes question God with, "Why me?" or, maybe it's, "Why not me?"

When I was going through this struggle, I had a friend who got pregnant after just one try at it. You'd better believe I was asking God "Why her? Why not me?" I eventually realized that kind of thinking would not change my circumstances. The only thing that could and would change my circumstances was God's Word...that's what I needed to be saying and praying instead of whining and complaining to Him. I needed to allow my hope to be fixed on God's solution and not on my burdensome circumstances.

God's power within us has given us everything we need for life. By knowing and standing on His precious promises, we are partakers or partners in His divine nature (2 Peter 1:3-4). Isn't that great to know? That's a reason to have hope! In other words, when we make it a point to read the Bible, learn His Word, and trust His promises, His promises to us are certain to make our lives successful in every area, even when it comes to having a baby.

Romans 5:1-2 says that we should expect God's glory to rise up within us and rejoice in the hope of His glory. When we do that, we won't feel as if we're fighting our battles by ourselves. We won't need to depend on our "self" to win; we'll depend on and rest in the greater power of God that is within us. With God on our side, we're not fighting this battle against infertility alone and we can be assured of victory.

Speak the Word: My hope is in God. I will not be made ashamed because of my hope. God has equipped me with everything I need for abundant life and victory.

More Encouragement: Psalm 39:7; Psalm 31:4; Psalm 16:9; 1 John 4:4

Dig Deeper: When do you find that you feel the most hopeful about your fertility? Why?

Pay Attention!

"My son, give attention to my words; Incline your ear to my sayings." ~Proverbs 4:20~

The thoughts we think repeatedly tend to eventually become the words we speak. Since our words shape our future, we really need to pay attention to what we're thinking. In other words, think about what you're thinking about!

The Bible tells us in Jeremiah 29:11 that God said the thoughts He thinks about us are positive and good. They are thoughts of peace and not of evil. His thoughts about us, which are expressed in His Word, give us a future with an outcome of hope. Does His explanation of His way of thinking indicate that God thinks you should be infertile and that you should forever remain that way? NO! He's thinking thoughts of fertility and abundance toward you!

God says that His thoughts are higher than our thoughts. This means there's room for improvement when it comes to our thought life. Instead of dwelling on the fact that another monthly menstrual cycle has started, or that you have a referral to yet another fertility specialist, choose a higher thought, a God-given thought.

Instead of wondering if you'll ever get pregnant, *choose* to think about something else. Fix your thoughts on things from God's Word that are lovely, true, pure, and praiseworthy (Philippians 4:8). That's thinking like Jesus thinks.

It just feels better when you think about good things, especially the things that God has said in His Word to bless you. It makes a significant difference in how you feel physically and emotionally when you dwell on things that are good and uplifting rather than those things that make you feel fearful and desperate.

Jesus has made a way for you to bring good things into your life and it starts with your thought life. Make the conscious effort to *pay attention* to what you're thinking about today and enjoy thinking about the good things God has for you.

Speak the Word: I pay attention to the words that God has spoken about my life. They are words of peace, wisdom and goodness. I am thankful that He blesses me with His words.

More Encouragement: Proverbs 7:24

Dig Deeper: Think about what you're thinking about. How can you apply God's words to your thoughts so that what you're thinking is aligned with His promises?

Confidence in Action #2

If you haven't already, pray together with your husband, asking God to make your uterus ready for impregnation, to have a healthy and safe pregnancy, and to deliver a healthy baby. Ask to become wise and godly parents from the beginning. And then, get together to pray prayers of thanksgiving often, trusting that God has heard your request and answered it (Psalm 138:3).

Reflections

_____

_____

_____

_____

_____

_____

_____

_____

_____

_____

_____

_____

_____

_____

_____

_____

_____

_____

This is War!

"For the weapons of our warfare are not carnal but mighty in God for pulling down strongholds."
~ 2 Corinthians 10:4 ~

Infertility is an attack. It is an attack from the devil. It is meant to steal your joy, kill your faith in God, and destroy your marriage (John 10:10).

Infertility is *not* sent from God in order to teach you some life lesson. Remember, only good gifts and perfect gifts come from God (James 1:17). He gives things that help us to have a full, abundant life. He has given us everything we need for abundant life and it's found in His Word (2 Peter 1:3).

Infertility's attack is not only on your body, but on your mind and spirit as well. It is meant to bring frustration, fear, disappointment, and even depression to your mind. It decreases the sexual enjoyment between you and your spouse because you become so focused on ovulation and perfect timing. You may sometimes say to yourself, "Is this the right time?" or, "We don't have much time!" Or it makes you wonder, "Where is the love?" The satisfaction of each sexual encounter can also decrease because of the repeated disappointment that may come each month as your menstrual cycle begins *again*.

Infertility can also affect your spirit. If you are a believer in Jesus Christ, you may very well begin to question whether

God has heard your cry for a baby, whether He really loves you, or whether He even exists.

Infertility can certainly be a strain on your finances. Going from doctor to doctor, having traditional and experimental tests and procedures done, can add up to a costly total. This acts as an additional source of stress in your marriage and in your body.

But God has given you victory over this enemy and every enemy that attacks you. His Word says that as a believer, you are *more* than a conqueror (Romans 8:37). "More than a conqueror" means that you have gained a *surpassing* victory through Jesus' victory!

I grew up in a sports-loving family so to me, being more than a conqueror means that I am on the team that romped over its enemy. I am more than a conqueror because Jesus is my teammate and He gave a thrashing, a clobbering, and an overwhelming defeat to *anything and everything* that does not promote abundant life. If you are a believer, then you are on Jesus' team, which means that you are *already* declared the victor, *not* a victim, even before you see the end of the battle against infertility.

So be encouraged. Put on the armor of God and fight against this attack (Ephesians 6:10-13). Pick yourself up, dust yourself off and STAND on the strength of the promises of God's Word, not on your own strength. Take action to win!

The only way to win is to use God's armor and weapons—meditating on His Word, singing songs of praise, expressing your gratitude to Him and spending time with Him in prayer. You may not see an immediate difference but your faith in God and His Word, mixed with patience, can change things.

When you make His Word an integral part of your life, His promises will cause you to win. When thoughts of doubt enter your mind, put them in their place (OUT of your mind!) by *speaking* His promises. When a doctor or someone else says something that makes you worry about whether you'll ever have a child, don't agree with those worrisome thoughts.

You are not forgotten nor defeated!

Speak the Word: I believe and do what God's Word says. I trust God because He's faithful, His Word is my truth and He will never fail to come through for me. I fight to maintain faith by using the weapons of God, not my own strength. My weapons are mighty through God. I use them to pull down the stronghold of infertility.

More Encouragement: Ephesians 6:10-18; 1 Corinthians 15:57-58

Dig Deeper: What's your **most** effective weapon of spiritual warfare?
*Affirming God's Word aloud
*Praying Scripture
*Singing songs of praise
*Praying in tongues
*Expressing gratitude in spite of the problem

*Other_____

It's a Take Down!

"Casting down imaginations, and every high thing that exalts itself against the knowledge of God, and bringing into captivity every thought to the obedience of Christ."
~ 2 Corinthians 10:5 ~

Y ou may think your circumstances of infertility are almost unbearable. But the Word tells us to have hope because every circumstance must bow its knee to the name of Jesus. His powerful name is above anything else (Philippians 2:9,10). As a believer in Him, you have the authority to use His name to take down those negative circumstances.

Make a decision to cast down those subtle reasonings that can stealthily and repeatedly slip into your mind. You are instructed in God's Word to cast down negative thoughts and to not dwell on them because they can become strongholds in your mind. You must not dwell upon those imaginations and thoughts that are hostile to or opposed to the Word of God.

Imagine that you are in a wrestling match. Your goal is to "take down" or to "cast down" your opponent. The same holds true with your thoughts. Demolish the thoughts that are constantly bombarding you about being childless. This will help you to keep from wavering in your faith. That's why the Word says to bring *all* your thoughts into captivity to the obedience of Jesus.

Choose to guard your mind and to consistently take down any fearful and negative thoughts. You do *not* have to tolerate them! Make a decision to allow the love and strength of Jesus to be the safe refuge for your thoughts.

Speak the Word: I cast down every thought I have which goes against the Word of God and I bring my thoughts into captivity to the obedience of Jesus.

More Encouragement: Deuteronomy 33:27; Psalm 94:19

Dig Deeper: What can you do to guard your thoughts so that negativity doesn't become (or continue to be) your normal way of thinking?

Faith-filled Sarah

" Because of faith, Sarah herself received physical power
to conceive a child, even when she was long past the age
for it, because she considered God Who had given her the
promise to be...true to His word."
~Hebrews 11:11 (AMP) ~

Sarah was the beloved wife of Abraham. She was over 90 years old when she got pregnant with her first child.

This was a miracle because Sarah had already gone through menopause (Genesis 18:11). Can you imagine giving birth at such a "mature" age?

Sarah must have still "had it going on" even in her old age because other men still desired her (Genesis 12:11-15, 20:2). She must have been doing a good job of taking care of herself through the years—an example all women should follow! But more than that, God blessed her with renewed youth, to look good and feel strong.

Even though Sarah had been barren (infertile) for an extremely long time, God promised Abraham that he would have a multitude of children. Many times, He reminded Abraham and Sarah of this promise (Genesis 13:16; 15:4, 5; 17:7, 15-17, 21; 18:10). Although God had repeatedly reminded them of His promise that they would have children, Sarah still had doubts. Even when God told them *when* the baby would be born, Sarah laughed and wondered "Shall I really bear a child when I'm so old?"

It's easy for us to slip into doubt too. Even though God may be giving us gentle reminders of His promises, we sometimes choose not to hold on until the fulfillment of His Word. That's when we have to do a self-check and encourage ourselves with what He has promised. Sarah later decided that God really was faithful to do what He had spoken. During the next year, just as God had said, she gave birth to a son, a son of promise. They named him Isaac.

Make a decision to view God as reliable, worthy of your trust and true to His Word. Be controlled and sustained by faith in Jesus' love for you. Confess God's promises as being true for your life. Have faith that He is not a respecter of persons (Acts 10:34). This means that what He did for Sarah He will do for you as you walk by faith in His unending love for you and not in fear of your current circumstances.

Determine to be faith-filled and to trust in the reliability and truthfulness of God's promises.

Speak the Word: I consider God to be true to His Word.

More Encouragement: Proverbs 30:5; Psalm 119:160

Dig Deeper: How often do you remind yourself that God's promises of fertility are for *you*? Is that often enough so that you stand strong in faith?

Put It in Good Hands

"Give all your worries and cares to God, for he cares about what happens to you."
~ 1Peter 5:7 (NLT) ~

Some years ago, I had a tendency to worry about things and needed to find a way to stop. I knew in my head that I should not worry. I knew that the Bible says to "cast all your cares on Him for He cares for you." But I just couldn't seem to shake this bad habit of worrying about a few things beyond my control!

I then heard a preacher define worry as having faith in what the devil was saying. I certainly did not want to have faith in anything the devil had a part of, so I began to seek God about how to stop worrying.

The devil "tells" you things by introducing thoughts and images into your mind. You then have to determine whether you'll accept that thought and review it over and over again (worry) or if you'll banish it right away.

Kenneth E. Hagin, a preacher of the gospel and great teacher of faith, gave an account of how sometimes he would be awakened in the middle of the night with a worrisome thought. Instead of continuing to think about it and lose sleep over it, he would simply whisper to the devil that he had already put that problem in God's hands. He would then instruct the devil to go take it up with God about that matter. Then he'd turn over and go back to sleep.

Genius! What great faith! What soldier-like execution of Jesus' command to have faith in God!

So I decided to start doing the same thing. I had to *repeatedly and consistently* respond in this way because the thoughts didn't just come once and then desist. They came repeatedly. And they didn't just come while I was sleep; they came in the middle of the day, while I was driving, when I was cooking dinner, even in the shower. I had to repeatedly respond with a verbal remark expressing my faith in God.

Eventually, those thoughts would stop but then new ones would come. And as a soldier of the Lord, I'd have to choose to fight again and not retreat from the battle in my mind. I had to focus my attention on God's truth, His power, and His love for me. I had to express my belief in Him by speaking with confidence in those things. As a result, I could consistently fight on, even though the bombardment of worrisome thoughts was evil's attempt to convince me to quit.

In this exercise of seeking God, He gave me a song. The song God gave me is now a tool that I use to remind myself to let Jesus handle my problems, situations, and issues. It is something I'd like to share with you and I hope it'll encourage you to trust God and put the issue of infertility, and any other problems in your life, in His hands.

It's in your hands Lord
It's in your hands
I don't worry about tomorrow
It's in your hands
I don't worry about today
'Cause I know you've made a way
It's in your hands Lord
It's in your hands
—Copyright © E. Colbert 2009

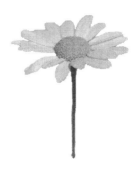

Speak the Word: I give all my worries to Jesus. I know He greatly loves me so I refuse to carry them because he died to remove them from my life.

More Encouragement: 1 Peter 5:7; Isaiah 10:27; Philippians 4:6

Dig Deeper: What do you visualize as you place your worries into God's hands?

Nothing But the Truth

"Sanctify them by Your truth. Your word is truth."
~ John 17:17 ~

Jesus said in His prayer in John 17 that God's Word is truth. Just what does that mean? Truth is defined as the *actual* state of a matter, an indisputable principle, conformity to reality, what is true in any matter, everything as it really was and is (Sources---Webster's 1828 dictionary, Dictionary.com). Thayer's Lexicon states that truth is the veracity of God keeping His promises.

Truth is on a higher level than facts. Truth is the way God sees things. Facts are the way man sees things. Facts are always subject to change. Truth is absolute and eternal. It does not ever change. It can however, change the facts that already exist. Truth is powerful! It can render something inoperative, depriving it of its power, and bringing it to naught (1 Corinthians 1:28).

If God's Word is truth and it is the *actual* state of a matter, then that implies that the facts of your present circumstance can be changed. By applying the pressure of the indisputable truth to the facts of your present circumstances, what is now visible in your physical world can be changed to line up with what God sees in the invisible spiritual world.

Have faith that God's Word is Truth. Have faith that He spoke it directly to you and for you. The answer, *your* answer can always be found in Him, no matter what the challenge is, no matter how impossible it may seem. God is always faithful to execute His Word. Nothing that He has EVER spoken has failed (1 Kings 8:56). You can count on His promises to change your situation.

Even though we can hear our words, we can't *see* them as we speak---they are invisible. The Bible says that it is the invisible that creates the visible. What's invisible can also change what's visible. This is not some hokey-pokey, mystical nonsense; this is how God operates!

The Bible declares that God created the heavens and the earth simply by speaking faith-filled words that described what he wanted to see. God changed the universe with words, which were spoken in faith. He uses the spiritual power of spoken words, which aren't seen, to nullify the existing natural things that are seen.

You can speak His powerful, living Word to change your circumstance of infertility. That Word is your truth, as seen from God's point of view. Confidently and consistently speak the truth, the whole truth and nothing but the truth!

Speak the Word: I speak God's Word in faith, because it is truth and is the one thing powerful enough to change my circumstances into what God wants them to be.

More Encouragement: Psalm 119:43, 142, 151; John 8:32; John 14:6

Dig Deeper: How can you *consistently* make God's Word your truth?

An Attitude of Gratitude

"Oh, give thanks to the LORD, for He is good! For His mercy endures forever."
~ 1 Chronicles 16:34 ~

When someone gives you a gift, do you leave it in their hands or do you take hold of it and pull it toward you? Most of us will grab it and receive it with a big grin on our face and delight in our eyes!

When you take possession of a gift, it becomes yours. You have become the owner of it. You can use it however you'd like. You also have the option to put it in a corner or on a shelf and never receive any benefit from being the new owner of it.

Long ago, I realized that the healing of my body was like a gift and I had not taken possession of it. So I purchased a pretty little gold cardboard gift box and set it on my dresser where I'd see it everyday. It was a visual and tactile reminder that I needed to take possession of what Jesus died for---my abundant life. So every time I'd see it or pick it up, I was reminded to say, "Thank you God, I receive my healing."

Saying "thank you" is an important part of receiving. Not only are you being polite, you're also telling the giver that you're grateful for what they've taken the time to provide or do for you. In my case, I was telling God that I was grateful for His love and for the healing He had already provided for me through the body of Jesus. I chose to have an attitude of gratitude even when I was still experiencing infertility. I chose to thank God for His goodness, for His dynamic healing power working in me, and for His unconditional love.

By saying "thank you", you're also telling yourself that you have taken possession of something. You are reminding yourself that you have received the gift and taken ownership of it. When you hear yourself say "thank you" over and over again with genuineness, you begin to build up your confidence. You're building up your faith!

Romans 10:17 says, "Faith comes by hearing, and hearing." Hearing yourself say to God, "Thank you for a healthy baby", *even in the midst of infertility*, is a means of keeping yourself focused on Him and His solution to the problem. You are reinforcing within your mind that you are strengthened and receiving Life from Him. Stay focused on God, the Giver of good gifts by giving Him thanks, right where you are.

> *Prayer for Today:* Father God, I come to you today giving you thanks and praise for Your faithfulness in my life. Thank you that as I choose to receive Your Word, it works to give me abundant life and it strengthens my soul. Help me to keep my heart and mind focused on You. In Jesus' Name. Amen.

Speak the Word: God is good and I am thankful that He is faithful to me.

More Encouragement: Psalm 84:11; Psalm 89:24

Dig Deeper: How do you show appreciation to God?

No Condemnation

"There is therefore now no condemnation to those who are in Christ Jesus, who do not walk according to the flesh, but according to the Spirit." ~ Romans 8:1 ~

A lot of us suffer from invisible wounds---those emotional wounds that take seemingly forever to heal.

Many things cause invisible wounds. One cause that's not openly talked about very much is abortion. Have you ever had an abortion? If you have, my prayer for you is that the resulting, and possibly still lingering, emotional wounds would be healed. The physical scars within your body are not the only wounds that take time to heal. Many women suffer through emotional wounds (guilt, lack of trust in men, self-condemnation) for decades after having an abortion. There are also spiritual wounds that need to be healed—wounds that cause you to pull away from God, to stop praying, to think that infertility may be your punishment. Maybe you've stopped believing that God is on your side.

The good news is that an abortion, or even multiple abortions, will not cause God to pull away from you or to stop loving you. The Bible says in Romans 8:35-39 that nothing that we have done or will ever do is able to separate us from the love of God, if we are a believer in Jesus Christ. It's time to stop holding on to the guilt and self-condemnation. It's time to be free and enjoy the liberty

Jesus died to give you. Jesus knows *everything* about you and He *still* loves you.

He chooses, out of love, to not condemn any of us. He chose at the cross to be judged and condemned on our behalf so that we don't ever have to be judged or condemned. Romans 8:1-2 assures us that there is no more condemnation to anyone who is in union with Jesus. If you are a believer, you've been made free from condemnation for your past acts. Isn't that good news? A new power is in operation! It's the power of LIFE, which comes by asking Jesus into your heart. It's time to stop holding onto past mistakes. God doesn't hold on to them, why should you?

God has qualified you through the blood of Jesus to forever be able to receive His blessings. When He looks at you as a believer in Christ, He sees the blood of Jesus, not your failings, your shortcomings, or your mistakes. Ask God to take everything that you have allowed to hold you back from receiving the *fullness* of His love and the complete healing of your emotional wounds.

Allow His love to be poured out on you like oil, anointing every part of you--from head to toe, inside and out. It's time to give yourself permission to receive God's unconditional love, forgiveness and grace. After all, Jesus' love for you was what prompted Him to die for you and allow you to forever have *His* right standing with God the Father. Let Him love you back to wholeness.

It's also time to forgive yourself. It's time to allow your born-again spirit to rule over your mind and thoughts so that you can live with confidence that you are free of condemnation and anything that works to keep you in bondage to your past. This is the time…be free NOW!

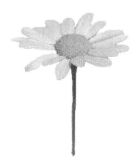

Speak the Word: Because of Jesus' love and His righteousness that He gave me, I am not condemned; I am redeemed and forgiven. Therefore I live freely in the abundance of His grace.

More Encouragement: John 3:16,17; Hebrews 8:10,12; Psalm 103:10-12; Romans 8:33

Dig Deeper: In what areas of your life do you most frequently hear yourself saying self-deprecating words? What causes you to do so? How will you change that?

Effective Prayer

"For the eyes of the Lord are over the righteous, and his ears are open unto their prayers." ~ 1 Peter 3:12 ~

I remember praying many times, "God, please let me be pregnant this time." It was usually while standing in my bathroom, right before I used a pregnancy home test kit. It was *not* a very effective prayer.

Thankfully, God is wonderfully merciful and He started me on a journey of learning more about prayer and how to pray effectively to get results that I desired. I had to learn more—what I had been doing was not working! James 5:16 reveals that the fervent, effective prayer of a righteous person produces much. Well, my prayer was fervent, but it was not effective. It had no power. Begging God to do something was not working!

God has a system. And when we live within His system, we get excellent results! God's system requires that we trust in His love for us. It necessitates that we have faith in Him (Hebrews 11:6), that we believe His Word, speak His Word, and put action to what we believe. His system requires speaking His Word, not only as a "confession" but also in our normal conversation. Our conversational words with others throughout the day should not negate what we've confessed as God's promise to us.

For instance, I would find myself complaining over and over again to Freeman or one of my other friends about not being pregnant yet and then, every month, asking God,

"Why am I not pregnant yet?" Fortunately, I learned that what you say over and over again is typically what you believe deep down inside yourself, in your heart. So I had to make the conscious effort to change what I was saying to my husband, my friends, co-workers and others. I had to start saying and continue to say that I believed that God intended for Freeman and me to have a baby. I had to persevere in praying His Word and trusting the Word to do its work (Psalm 107:20).

As my conversations and prayers began to line up with God's system, I began to see results. Listen to what you are saying in your prayers and your conversations with others. Make sure it lines up with what you want! Your determination, in praying His Word and in resting in His grace, is an expression of your faith in His goodness. It's the means of opening the door for His power to move in your life and bring the results you desire.

Speak the Word: I thank God for His Word. I believe it and I speak it in both my conversations and my prayers.

More Encouragement: Proverbs 18:21; Psalm 102:1

Dig Deeper: What is an *effective* prayer? Write one here about your fertility.

_____

_____

_____

_____

_____

Yes, God *Still* Heals!

"He sends forth His word and heals them and rescues them
from the pit and destruction."
~ Psalm 107:20 ~

I am living proof that God is still in the healing business. After hearing from my gynecologist that he was sending me to a specialist to determine why I could not get pregnant, I thought that childlessness maybe our permanent "condition". In looking for a reason for why I was not yet pregnant, some of my test results prompted him to tell my husband and me that we may never be able to conceive a child.

Fortunately, we were members of a church where the pastor believed in the power of prayer. He and his wife taught the church family that prayer could change things. So Freeman and I began to pray more frequently after hearing the doctor's opinion. I began to keep a journal where I would write various scripture verses that dealt with the power of God's Word. I didn't know it at the time, but I was putting into practice what Proverbs 4:20-22 says: *"Pay attention to God's words. Keep reading them and thinking about them. Why? Because they bring life to anyone who finds them, and they bring healing and health for their entire body and mind"* (my paraphrase).

I kept looking for and finding more scriptures that would build up my faith. I would write them out in my journal and add a note under each one about how I understood its application to our circumstance of infertility. In other words, I would paraphrase it like you read the passage from Proverbs 4 above, so that I could understand it better and apply it to my life. As I got deeper into the Word, I found that God blessed me—this was the only way I was able to have some level of peace through more months of not conceiving.

Because I was focusing more on Him, I was not so focused on the inability to get pregnant. I also found that doing this gave me more confidence in not only God's ability, but also His *willingness* to heal whatever was wrong with my body so that I could conceive. Where there is confidence, there is expectation. Where there is expectation, there is hope. Where there is hope, there is an inner image of something coming. I had to hold on to that confidence in God for me to be healed, pregnant, and deliver a healthy baby.

Speak the Word: My confidence and hope are in God. I put my attention to His Words. They bring life, health, and healing to my body.

More Encouragement: Psalm 103:1-4; Psalm 119:50; Matthew 8:17

Dig Deeper: Where will you choose to place your focus— on your struggle with infertility or on God's love for you and His willingness to heal you?

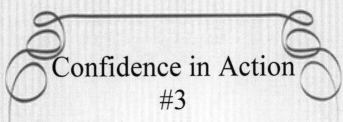

Confidence in Action
#3

Begin to *prepare* your body:

Get a health check-up from your doctor or health care professional. If you already have weight-caused health issues, get a plan to help you get to a healthy weight.

Begin to take prenatal vitamins, especially a formula that includes folic acid.

Eliminate sources of caffeine in what you eat and drink. Some studies have shown that caffeine intake may affect fertility.

Eat more healthy foods---leafy vegetables, fruit, whole grains, and lean protein.

Eliminate smoking cigarettes/marijuana and drinking all alcoholic beverages.

Begin an exercise routine to strengthen your muscles. Learn how to do Kegel exercises and do them consistently to strengthen your pelvic muscles for a vaginal delivery.

Reflections

Tired of "Trying"?

"And they were both naked, the man and his wife, and were not ashamed." ~Genesis 2:25 ~

Infertility can take all the polish and shine off of lovemaking and turn it into a dull, forced, functional act of baby making.

Have you reached a point where you're asking yourself, "What happened to the intimacy?" or "What happened to the fun?"

When we became so focused on charting my basal temperature to find my time of ovulation and the best time of fertility, sex eventually became work. We had to manage logistics, revise schedules, etc. Even if we were tired from everything else in our busy lives, it didn't matter. We *had* to "do it," since it could be another 28 days before that egg was in the right spot to receive a sperm.

Sex is supposed to be an intimate time of sharing your body with your spouse. A time of "two becoming one." A time of expressing love in a physical way, even a time of releasing stress. But it can quickly become a *stress-producer* instead, when you're constantly wondering during that time together, "Will I get pregnant this time?" Nobody wants to go through another month wondering if it worked. Nobody wants to answer "No" again to the repeated question from others, "Are you pregnant yet?"

If this has become your reality, as mundane as it may have become, you still must perform the sex act in order to make a baby! So determine ways that you can stay upbeat about continually "trying", even if it does not result in immediate pregnancy. Ask God for wisdom on how to keep the romance alive and meaningful. Encourage yourself and your spouse. Plan fun date nights or weekends away from home, if possible. Increase moments of intimacy during the rest of the month so that you still experience the joy of lovemaking without the stress of "baby-making".

I know it can be very difficult to maintain that joy, but you must decide now that the health of your marriage will always be more important than any other factors in your life together. You'll want your child to enjoy the security of a life lived with a mom and dad who are committed to one another no matter what.

Speak the Word: I submit my marriage to the Lord and allow His joy to be expressed in my life through intimacy with my husband.

More Encouragement: Genesis 2:24, 25; Song of Solomon 7:6, 10-12

Dig Deeper: What can you do to add some "spark" to lovemaking the next time you're intimate with your husband?

The Power Tool of Praise

"Save us, O LORD our God, and gather us from among the heathen, to give thanks unto thy holy name, and to triumph in thy praise." ~ Psalm 106:47 ~

Praise is strength!
Praise is a source of power!
Praise is a mighty tool!

Psalm 8:2 states that praise *"stills"* the enemy. In other words, it causes his work to cease, to desist from activity. Imagine that! You, through praising God, can restrain the enemy (the devil) and put an end to the momentary battle going on in your mind. Try it right now, even if it feels awkward for you to speak a few words of praise out loud to God.

When you're feeling like giving in to the thought that infertility is your permanent condition, speak words of praise instead. When your thoughts are of discouragement, impatience, and doubt, speak words of praise—think about what victories God has already brought you through in other areas of you life. Verbally thank Him for them. Tell Him how good He is. He's not looking for your accolades to make Him feel good or puffed up. Rather, He has ordained praise as a tool for your use on your way to victory. It puts your mind on what He can do instead of what you can't do in your own power. Tell Him how you trust Him. Tell Him how He is the One who has *already* given you victory over infertility. That's praise!

Now you may be thinking, He hasn't given me victory—I'm not pregnant. Well, banish that thought! Right this minute, tell yourself, out loud, that God has indeed given you victory over infertility. Believe that it's done. *Praise Him in advance* of its manifestation. Jesus finished the work and guaranteed the covenant by giving His body and blood on your behalf. That's why you have authority to use the power tool of praise.

Everyday, take time to verbally praise Jesus for His love, His uncompromising character and for all He's done. You can even *sing* your words of praise to Him. The more you do this, the more you'll see your confidence in Him increase. You'll soon be saying in the face of infertility, "Hallelujah anyhow!"

Speak the Word: Praise is what I do because I know that Jesus has done *everything* necessary to give me a life of overflowing abundance.

More Encouragement: Psalm 145:21; Psalm 112:1,2; Psalm 117:1, 2

Dig Deeper: What are some ways you can begin to "praise God in advance" for the things you've asked Him to do or provide?

Put Pen to Paper

"And the Lord answered me and said, write the vision and make it plain upon tablets, that he may run that reads it."
~ Habakkuk 2:2 ~

Regularly writing your thoughts about overcoming infertility can help you to keep track of your mindset. This enables you to more quickly make adjustments if you get off course and begin to have a pity-party. Writing your thoughts can assist you in keeping the faith for getting pregnant and delivering a healthy baby.

The Bible tells us to write our thoughts, our hopes, and our dreams. But we're not to stop there. We're to *use* what we've written about them. In the scripture from Habakkuk, the word "run" means to move quickly and to take action. So get a notepad or a journal and describe how you see yourself as an overcomer of infertility. Use very descriptive words that help you see a picture in your mind. Give details of how you see yourself fertile, pregnant, delivering a healthy baby, and being a wise, loving parent.

It would be a good idea to write out corresponding scriptures as well. Write the ones that encourage you, that build up your faith in Jesus, that point to motherhood as not only a possibility but as a reality. You could also include scriptures that remind you of God's love for you and the authority and dominion you have in life because of Jesus.

Consider asking God to show you a particular scripture that will begin to shape your child's life and destiny. Write it in your journal and begin to speak it now, even before your baby is formed in your womb (Jeremiah 1:5). Speak it throughout the coming months of pregnancy and continue to do so after the baby is born.

I'm grateful to have my journals to look back through. They are a source of encouragement and a measuring stick of how much I've grown in the struggles of life. Perhaps most importantly, they are a testimonial to the goodness of God and how running with His Word delivered me from infertility and moved me into a life of "Mommyhood".

Speak the Word: I make a written record of what I envision that God will do in my life so that I can take action according to His Word.

More Encouragement: Habakkuk 2:3; Proverbs 29:18

Dig Deeper: What are 3 of your favorite scriptures about God's love for you? Write them out in a journal, or on an index card, or on sticky note and refer to them often.

The Supply Chain of Grace

"Grace and peace be multiplied unto you through the knowledge of God, and of Jesus our Lord." ~ 2 Peter 1:2 ~

In God's supply chain of grace, there is no middleman we must go through. We can go to Him and receive from Him directly, without the delay that a middleman causes in a typical transaction.

God has hands (Psalm 92:4) and they are open because He is willing to freely give good gifts and perfect gifts to all. He wants to provide us with a constant flow of grace as we make requests of Him. He is the supplier of all our desires. He is willing for us to take from Him as much as we want.

God has arms (Deuteronomy 33:27) and they are strong and far-reaching. What do His hands and arms have to do with anything you're going through now? Those loving hands and strong arms supply the abundant grace you need to make it *through* infertility so that you don't get stuck *in* it. God is ready and able to help you turn things around right now. He cares about you and is not only able but also willing to get you through this.

God also has ears (Psalm 27:7) and they hear with excellent clarity. When you call to Him, He hears you. The Bible says in 1 John 5:14 that when we ask anything according to His will, He hears us. His Word, the Bible, *is* His will. So if you can find it in His Word and you ask Him for it in Jesus' name, you can have confidence that He has heard you. Verse 15 goes on to say that if we know that He has heard us, then we can know that we have what we have asked of Him. The key here is to *ask according to His Word.* Have faith that His promises in His Word are for you personally. He has already provided and supplied what He has said in His Word in the finished work of Jesus on the cross. It's up to you to accept it, to believe it, to receive it, to take hold of it and not let go until you see it manifested.

God desires to abundantly supply you with His grace. There is no limit to His powerful grace! He desires to show Himself strong on your behalf. His grace is sufficient for you to overcome, conquer, and destroy the enemy of infertility. Because of His grace, as you hold on to His promises and don't allow doubt or unbelief to dictate to you what you should do, He will always cause you to triumph (2 Corinthians 2:14)!

How much of His grace are you willing to receive? Get in on this marvelously abundant supply of grace. He offers even more than what you need. His supply of grace to you never runs out!

Speak the Word: I am growing in my knowledge of Jesus and His love for me. His wonderful grace is being multiplied in my life and it never runs out.

More Encouragement: John 1:16; 2Corinthians 12:9; 2Chronicles 16:9; Ephesians 3:20

Dig Deeper: When have you experienced God's grace so abundantly that it seemed to pleasantly overwhelm you?

Joy

"...for the joy of the Lord is your strength."
~ Nehemiah 8:10 ~

The joy that comes from the Lord strengthens us in *every* situation, even the most stressful ones!
I remember there were moments when I was feeling lonely, tired of suffering with infertility's emotional drain, and sometimes feeling afraid of my future. Those were the moments I had to remind myself to choose to make an attitude adjustment and get to a joyful frame of mind.

You too must choose to let joy rise to the surface of your mind so it can strengthen you by snuffing out fear and all those depressing emotions.

What are some ways you can stir up joy within you?
- Remember that God the Father loves you just like He loves Jesus.
- Sing an uplifting song.
- Say what you're grateful for. Write them in a "thankfulness diary".
- Praise God for how He is strengthening you.
- Read about other women who have overcome infertility.
- Read Bible verses that encourage you (here are a few to get you started):
    - Psalm 16:11
    - 2 Peter 1:3
    - Psalm 5:11

- o Deuteronomy 28:4,11
- o Romans 15:13
- Remind yourself, by frequently telling yourself out loud, that God wants to bless you in ways above and beyond what you're capable of imagining. (Ephesians 3:20)

Be open to what God has to say to you so that your joy will be *full*. Meditate on His Word and pray, because the Bible says that in His presence is the fullness of joy. Open your heart to Him and allow His joy that He gives to bless you with strength spiritually, physically, and on some days most importantly, emotionally. Thank God for His *fullness* of joy in your life!

Speak the Word: I choose to rejoice in the Lord daily. The joy of the Lord strengthens me.

More Encouragement: Psalm 32:11; Psalm 89:15-18

Dig Deeper: What can you say aloud to yourself everyday to bolster the level of joy you experience in Him?

Life and Death are in the Power of *Your* Tongue

"Death and life are in the power of the tongue."
~ Proverbs 18:21 ~

Proverbs 18:21 reveals that our tongue holds the power of life and death. This means that the words that we say are powerful!

Our words actually contain the power to *promote* life or to *promote* death. God allows us to have free will to choose what we will say, which ultimately means that we get to choose "life" for our circumstances or "death" for our circumstances.

In the circumstance of childlessness, we definitely want to speak LIFE--- life to our bodies, our emotions, our marriage and even our finances!

Allow God to fill your mouth with *good* things daily (Psalm 103:5):

- Declare that you are a child of God because of your faith in Jesus Christ (Galatians 3:26)
- Declare that you are loved unconditionally by God the Father, in the same way that He loves Jesus (John 17:23)
- Declare that you reside in His circle of blessing (Psalm 25:13, Living Bible Version)

- Declare that you rest in Him and enjoy His peace that surpasses all understanding (Philippians 4:7)
- Declare that God's grace is sufficient in all your times of need (2 Corinthians 12:9)
- Declare that God is good and will never leave you nor turn His back on you (Hebrews 13:5)
- Declare that you are a partaker of His blessings. Your body is blessed, your mind is blessed, your marriage is blessed, and your children are blessed. (Deuteronomy 28:1-14; Galatians 3:13,14,29)
- Declare victory over infertility and childlessness because you are in Christ (1 Corinthians 15:57)

Find other scriptures that relate to your circumstances and speak them with confidence because God's words are spiritual containers that carry power!

Speak the Word: I choose to consciously speak words of life, victory and blessing throughout each day.

More Encouragement: Psalm 141:3; Proverbs 12:18; Psalm 49:3

Dig Deeper: What do you say about God? Are your everyday conversations tinged with love and gratitude or blame, doubt, and negativity?

Confidence in Action #4

Use what I call "the Holy BUT" in your everyday conversations. You can say, "I may not be pregnant "BUT" God said that none shall be barren (Exodus 23:26) and that includes me". His Truth is stronger than your fact. Truth is powerful and never changes. God's Truth never fails. God's truth can actually change your facts of life. What's God's Truth? It's His Word of love and grace toward you (John 17:17). God's Word doesn't change but it does change how you see yourself and your circumstances. It is absolute—you can count on it!

Reflections

_____

_____

_____

_____

_____

_____

_____

_____

_____

_____

_____

_____

_____

_____

_____

_____

_____

Thankfulness

*"Then I will praise God's name with singing, and I will
honor him with thanksgiving."*
~ Psalm 69:30 (NLT) ~

An entry that I had written in one of my old journals was dated 11/26/86, and was just a simple list of things I was thankful for that day.

It started out with some of the "usual" things—good health, a good husband, a nice home, friends, etc. What stood out most to me were these two items that I had included in the list:

- *A baby that is to come next year*
- *Children*

Keep in mind, I was not pregnant on 11/26/86 and had already been told by the doctor that I may never have children. It's interesting to look back and realize that even as I was in the midst of the battle against infertility I could choose to be thankful for a child.

A subsequent entry I wrote in that journal was a love note to me from God after spending some time in prayer with Him. I'd like to share part of it with you:

"You must believe, when you pray, that I will answer your prayers. You've reached the point where the baby will come next year. You'll bring

him up in the way he should go for I've called him already. Be still in Me and receive the blessings. Don't worry, I'm with you."

That entry was dated 1/25/87. Our son Nathan was born in June 1988. Isn't God good?

Many years later, I can see how being thankful is important. Writing on paper what I expected and expressing gratitude for it before I could see it was a part of how I received the blessing of a child and, eventually, the blessing of a total of three beautiful children. And I'm glad to say that I'm *still* thankful for each of them!

As I look back, I believe thankfulness, in advance of the manifestation of pregnancy, played an important role in our prayers being answered. The Bible says in Philippians 4:6 (AMP): "Do not fret or have any anxiety about anything, but in every circumstance and in everything, by prayer and petition [definite requests] *with thanksgiving*, continue to make your wants known to God."

Make the choice to be thankful to God *now* for what you're expecting to manifest in your future.

Speak the Word: I give honor to God by giving Him thanks for all that He has done and for all that He will do in my life.

More Encouragement: Colossians 4:2; 1 Chronicles 16:8-12

Dig Deeper: Before you go to bed tonight, write 3 things (big or small) that you're grateful for from today.

Let It Be For Me

"Then Mary said, "Behold the maidservant of the Lord! Let
it be to me according to your word." And the angel
departed from her." ~ Luke 1:38 ~

I have always been part of a family that enjoyed sports.
My dad played football in college and my closest
cousins played football and basketball. So it's no
surprise that I'm still in a family of sports enthusiasts. My
husband and sons were athletes in school. I enjoy attending
and watching football and basketball games with my
husband and children.

Football can be analogous to life in many ways and can
even be applied to what you may be experiencing with
infertility. One of the most important positions on a football
team is that of a receiver. He's the one that runs when the
ball is snapped and catches the ball when his quarterback
throws it to him. The quarterback always has a plan, a
vision, as to where he expects the receiver to be when he
throws the ball to him. If the receiver is not where the
quarterback expects him to be, if he's out of position, he
can't catch the ball.

We are much like that receiver. If we're "out of position",
it's likely we won't get to "catch" the blessings that God
has envisioned for us to receive. How do you make sure
you're "in position"? Release your faith in response to
God's love for you and to the promises found in His Word!
That's what Mary did when the angel told her that God
intended for her to become a mother to Jesus. Her response

was "Let it be as you have said." Mary did not know how it was going to happen, nor did she know when, but she made a decision to trust God. That decision to trust Him put her "in position" to receive what God had already promised her. Her miracle was in her mouth! Her trust, faith, and *words* connected her to God's supernatural realm where "nothing shall be impossible." (Luke 1:37)

Similarly, releasing *your* faith by trusting in and speaking the Word of God will also put you in position to receive. So take action—tell God, "Be it unto me according to your Word." There are instances in the Bible where it tells us of an event that will definitely happen simply because "the mouth of the Lord hath spoken it." So find scriptures in His Word that you can stand on as you seek to overcome childlessness. Trust that if God said it and you believe it, it shall be.

Hook up to His power so this natural realm---your senses, feelings and doctors' reports---does not limit your circumstances. Be like Jesus, communicate and be in union with God through words and prayers of faith. In spite of how impossible having a baby appears to be right now, believe that nothing is impossible because you have chosen to be a receiver, connected to the vision and power of God.

Speak the Word: Whatever God has said in His Word about my situation, I believe it and receive it...so be it!

More Encouragement: John 3:27; Matthew 21:22; Matthew 9:22

Dig Deeper: When do you feel out of position to receive from God? What corrective action do you take?

Victory

"For whatever is born of God overcomes the world. And this is the victory that has overcome the world—our faith."
~ *1 John 5:4* ~

Just as our country's soldiers fight on our behalf against an enemy, when they win, the entire country shares in the victory. Every citizen gets to say that the nation was victorious even though only a few actually fought the battle. It's the same way for us in spiritual battles, with Jesus as our defender.

Dealing with infertility *is* a spiritual battle as well as a physical, mental, and emotional one. But Jesus has already fought against the enemy AND WON (Colossians 2:14,15)! So we, as believers in Him, get to rest in His grace and share in His victory. We get to say to infertility, "I am victorious over you through Jesus Christ!"

Believe that God's Word is *the* Truth. Have faith that He spoke it directly to you and that it is *for* you and not against you. The answer, *your* answer, can always be found in Him, no matter what the challenge is, no matter how impossible it may seem. Because of His strength and unchanging love, God longs for you to walk in victory by allowing Him to be there for you as the Answer to every problem you face, even infertility.

Dig into the Word for yourself. Listen for Jesus to speak His wisdom to you for your specific circumstances through His Word and allow God's solution, His Truth, to bring you out victoriously. Speak it out loud as a confident affirmation. You will see the enemy called "infertility" turn tail and retreat, as you believe the Word's power to manifest change in your life.

Speak the Word: I have faith in the Word of God and I am assured of victory through Jesus!

More Encouragement: John 16:33; 1 Chronicles 29:11-13

Dig Deeper: What are some ways that you benefit from the victory Jesus has provided for you?

Speak to the Mountain

"For assuredly, I say to you, whoever says to this mountain,
'Be removed and be cast into the sea,' and does not doubt
in his heart, but believes that those things he says will be
done, he will have whatever he says." ~Mark 11:23~

Jesus instructs us in Mark 11:22-23 to have faith in God, to speak to the mountain or problem (in this instance, infertility) without doubting, and to believe that what we've spoken in faith will come to pass. Speaking out loud to the problem of infertility may feel a bit weird at first. But Jesus said that the mountain would have to move out of the way when spoken to in faith. So if you follow God's encouraging instructions by *consistently* speaking His Word to that "mountain" of infertility, that adverse circumstance must give in to the pressure brought by God's Word.

Here are some good reasons to believe and speak the words that God has spoken:

- His Word is forever settled, established, and it stands strong and erect. Psalm 119:89
- God is alert and active to perform His Word. Jeremiah 1:12
- He will not alter what He has spoken. Psalm 89:34
- God has promised and will never go back on His Word. Isaiah 45:23 (See the Living Bible Translation for special emphasis.)

Speak the Word to that mountain of infertility. When we hear ourselves speaking it, it helps us to stay connected to Jesus and enables us to walk in joy and blessing. Speak the Word, for in the beginning was the Word and in the end, the Word of God will remain standing when all else has failed you in this struggle against infertility. God wants to inundate you with His grace and His goodness. Choose to remain connected to Him through His Word and watch the blessings flow.

Speak the Word: I believe that God loves me and is willing to perform His Word on my behalf.

More Encouragement: Matthew 21:18-22

Dig Deeper: When do you find it easiest to speak to the mountain of infertility? What specifically do you say to it?

You Are Not Forgotten

"For He Himself has said, "I will never leave you nor forsake you." ~ Hebrews 13:5 ~

Remember what it was like as a kid to be left out when playing with your friends? Remember the anguish you felt when you didn't fit in while everyone else did or had something that you didn't? Infertility can make us tap into those same emotions as an adult, except on a much more intense and consequential level.

But, there's good news! You are not forgotten! God has not forgotten about you or the situations you find yourself in. He is willing to supply everything you need. His supply is more than you can take—He'll never run out of what you need. He'll never run out on you. He has not forgotten about you, your situation, or your cry for His help.

The Lord is always mindful of you. He always has you on His mind by thinking good thoughts toward you, by providing His grace, His favor, and His mercy everyday. In Jeremiah 29:11, God says, "I know the thoughts that I think towards you, says the Lord, thoughts of peace, and not of evil, to give you an expected end."

The only thing that God forgets is your sin. When you receive Jesus and repent of your sin, God says that He forgets it and removes it from us as far as the east is from the west (Psalm 103:12). Jesus died so that you benefit from *His* obedience to God. He prayed for your protection.

He prayed for you to live your life in the authority that was given to you through Him.

Jesus endured suffering, shame and a horrible death just for you. He endured it all so you wouldn't have to.

He did it all because He loves *you*. How could He possibly forget about *you*?

Speak the Word: Jesus said that He is always with me. He is ever mindful of me and will never leave me.

More Encouragement: Joshua 1:5; Jeremiah 50:5; Psalm 115:12

Dig Deeper: What is it that reassures you in your lowest moments that God loves you?

Be Expectant, Not Desperate

"It is good that one should hope and wait quietly for the salvation of the LORD."
~ Lamentations 3:26 ~

T here's a big difference between being desperate and being expectant in life's situations. When I was told that chances were great that I'd never have a baby and needed to begin considering tests and treatments for infertility, it was easy for desperation to quickly begin to creep in.

Desperation comes when you dwell on the likelihood of negative circumstances in your life never changing, of infertility never being reversed. You become desperate to find a solution, no matter the cost, the pain, or loss of intimacy. Desperation's companions are recklessness and aimlessness. They can make you feel that you're losing control of life's circumstances, and can make you seek out possibly unwise solutions that you'd never consider otherwise. It begins to gnaw away at your hope and eventually, if left unchecked, it can devour all the hope you've ever had of having a baby. Hope is that inner image that you hold on to, the image generated by God's promises. *When hope is lost, your faith no longer has a mission to accomplish.*

How do you move from being desperate to being expectant of good things, and as a result, having your hope renewed? Begin to search God's Word for a *reason* to hope. Jesus said that His Word is Truth (John 17:17) and truth is the only thing that can set you free from desperation and discouragement (John 8:32). Then you'll have reason to look forward to your circumstances changing because every promise in God's Word is a spirit-generated Word and is also life-generating. So make sure as you're confessing and speaking the Word that you confess it in faith, not desperation.

Have confidence as you speak the Word, knowing God the Father loves you just as He loves Jesus (John 17:23). Speak it with the anticipation and expectancy that God has done something about this circumstance of infertility. Instead of wondering, "What if He doesn't come through and answer my prayer with a 'yes'?" say to the source of that doubt, the devil, "What if God *does* come through?" Be like the farmer in James 5:7 who waits eagerly and patiently for the harvest. He doesn't fret about the seeds he's planted. He trusts that there will be seed germination, plant growth, and a harvest.

There are many seasons in life where we must wait. But if we wait with a hopeful and positive outlook, we won't fret or get anxious. Wait with an expectancy of God's favor to make you an overcomer of infertility.

By speaking and believing God's Word with expectancy, you allow the Spirit of God to rekindle hope inside of you. Allow His promises to light a fire of hope!

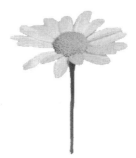

Speak the Word: I wait with patience and eagerness because my hope is in you Lord. I expect your Word to come to pass in my life.

More Encouragement: Lamentations 3:21-26; Hebrews 6:19

Dig Deeper: When are you most likely to experience a hope-filled outlook about your life? How can you sustain that?

Blessed Is She That Believed

*"I would have lost heart, unless I had believed that I would
see the goodness of the LORD in the land of the living."*
~ Psalm 27:13 ~

When we believe what God has said, we can be
sure that it shall come to pass. The message from
God to the Virgin Mary included an assurance
that there would be a performance of what God said. God's
Word always has action as a companion. When God
speaks, things happen!

Numerous times in the Old Testament, we see things
happened because "the mouth of the Lord had spoken it"
(Isaiah 40:5, 58:14). God doesn't waste His words. They
have power and they make things happen when someone
hears and believes what He has said.

When Freeman and I finally and truly believed God's Word
about there being no barrenness in us and that we would be
fruitful and multiply, we had a peace within us that a baby
would be born to us. It took trusting that what God said was
true and that it was for our situation. It took resting in His
grace He poured out to us through His Word.

Trusting in what God said meant we could rest from all the
anxiety we had been feeling for months. Even as people
encouraged us and prayed for us, I found myself always
wondering if it was *ever* going to happen. I had that thought

less frequently as I put myself in that place of rest --- resting in that peace found only in Jesus.

A friend of mine suggested that I search the scriptures for examples of women who had been infertile and then gave birth to a child. I followed her advice and found there were so many! Sarah, Abraham's wife, was not the only one.

Each of those women reached a point where they had to rest in God, trusting that He would do what He said. To read their stories was a great source of encouragement and I'm sure if you do the same, you'll find yourself moving to a greater level of peace and confidence about having victory over infertility.

Speak the Word: I believe that I continually see the goodness of God demonstrated in my life.

More Encouragement: Luke 1:45; Psalm 23:6

Dig Deeper: Will you make a decision to believe God's promises of fertility, cutting off any options that cause doubt and unbelief? How will you rest in knowing that He is able *and willing*?

The Value of Friends

"The heartfelt counsel of a friend is as sweet as perfume and incense." ~ Proverbs 27:9 (NLT) ~

Sometimes, couples find themselves keeping the struggle of infertility a secret. They may feel as if no one would understand their struggle.

It would be easy for them to fear that they would be looked upon with pity. Dealing with infertility caused me to experience a wide variety of emotions, ranging from inadequacy to fear to shame. Thankfully, I had a friend who wrote me a note of encouragement to find women in the Bible who had overcome infertility in seemingly impossible circumstances.

I would encourage you and your spouse to discuss and agree about sharing your 'situation' with your pastor, a wise friend, or another couple that you *trust*. Open yourself to receive godly counsel, comforting words, and undergirding prayers.

My friend's note prompted me to learn more about these women's stories. I thought that maybe I could boost my level of hope by learning of their success over infertility. The exercise of searching the scriptures actually did more than just provide encouragement about overcoming infertility. It put me on a path that led to a love of searching the Word and finding promises that applied to many other areas of my life—health and healing, finances, marriage, and many more. It caused me to become Word-dependent.

It's important you surround yourself with people who will support you in this battle. Distance yourself from those who would discourage you. Your words and your thoughts are being shaped by what you choose to internalize from others. Your words and your thoughts will in turn shape what you'll live in your future. This matter is too important to allow anyone else to convince you that infertility is something that is beyond God's reach or too hard for Him to change.

God can use your friends in unexpected ways that can bring great joy and comfort to your life. I pray that you will value the godly friendships you have and will reap great benefit through their being used by God to encourage you.

Speak the Word: I am thankful that God provides friends who give me wise counsel and comfort. I surround myself with those who support me by giving me wise counsel and by speaking words of faith about my future.

More Encouragement: Proverbs 15:22; Proverbs 17:17; Proverbs 24:6

Dig Deeper: Which of your friends encourage you the most in this struggle? Send them a handwritten "Thank you" note.

Thou Shalt Not Fear!

*"For God has not given us a spirit of fear, but of power
and of love and of a sound mind."*
~ 2 Timothy 1:7 ~

Fear can be a gigantic foe in dealing with infertility. It haunted me daily through thoughts like "What if I never get pregnant?"

What do you fear most about infertility? Perhaps it's that it's lasted so long that you're already over 37 years of age and have been told that even if you got pregnant, you'd have a high-risk pregnancy. Or maybe you're embarrassed (which is a form of fear) that you and your husband are the only couple among your closest friends that haven't had a baby yet. Do you fear that you'll never have a baby? Well, STOP IT, because there's hope!

Fear is simply:
False
Evidence
Appearing
Real

Imagine if you were in a court setting, serving on a jury, hearing and being shown evidence that definitely points to the guilt of the defendant. You process that information given to you as being real, reliable, even truth. But then the defense attorney presents additional evidence, perhaps DNA test results that prove without a shadow of a doubt that the prosecutor's original evidence was false. Even though the original evidence was believable, it was not true--- it was actually false.

Now imagine that Satan is that prosecutor, presenting you with evidence so believable that even medical test results verify what he's saying—you're infertile. You feel your fear level increasing; you can even feel its effect in your body. But then Jesus steps up and tells you that Satan's evidence is false even though it appears real. Jesus would show you the Truth, which was written long before His birth, death and resurrection that said He had taken away ALL sickness and infirmity (Isaiah 53:3-5). He would reassure you of His love for you and His desire to pour out His goodness in your life.

Jesus would ask you to not fear and to believe that only His evidence is true and not Satan's. Then He'd tenderly and lovingly instruct you to have faith in Him and receive the inheritance of good health that He died to give you. Fear has no power when you're fighting the good fight of faith in Jesus Christ.

Fear believes in false evidence. Faith believes only in God's love and truth. **Whose report will you believe?**

Speak the Word: Jesus loves me and has not given me a spirit of fear but of power, love and a sound mind.

More Encouragement: Psalm 23:4; Isaiah 41:10; 1 John 4:16,18

Dig Deeper: What role does fear play in your thoughts and words? Has fear taken too much territory in your mind?

The Power of Communion

*"...Take, eat: this is my body which is broken for you: this
do in remembrance of me."*
~ 1 Corinthians 11:24 ~

Jesus commanded those who believe in Him to
frequently take part in the covenant meal because by
doing so, they fondly remember Him and His finished
work of grace. The covenant meal, or, communion as we
call it today, is a reminder of the sacrifice of Jesus' body
and blood on our behalf, as our substitute. It is also an
acknowledgement of the grace-exchange we can now make
with Him, because we receive Him as Savior.

The exchange we make is one where we give up our
weaknesses to God and take on His strengths as our own.
That's what covenant is all about—establishing a
commitment so strong that it cannot be broken, regardless
of how either party performs. Because God made this
covenant with Himself on our behalf, it is based only on
His performance and *His* strength. *It will never fail because
it is not based on our performance.* We get to benefit from
this unbreakable covenant because at His death, we as
believers in Jesus, became heirs to all He possessed.

Exodus 20:24 states when God is brought to our
remembrance, He will come and He will bless. Jesus
instructed us to take communion in order to bring Him to
our remembrance. This is not an instruction to do
something "in memory of" Him, as we would a dead
relative. Jesus is telling us to affectionately remember His

love that benefitted us in our body, mind, and spirit. His death and resurrection were great acts of love that live on for our benefit even through today.

As you continue this walk of faith to overcome infertility, consider taking communion at home as often as you think about it. Communion is not just a religious ritual that must be done within the confines of a church building nor is it required that a priest or a member of clergy always administer it. You can get your own crackers and juice and celebrate communion in your home. After all, the Last Supper took place in a home, not a synagogue or church. Jesus said to celebrate communion often (1 Corinthians 11:25). He knew that as we frequently remember Him and His love for us, we enable His grace to empower us and bless us.

In Luke 22:19, Jesus said His body was "given" for you. That means He was delivering His body for your benefit and use. He presented Himself for you to literally take advantage of all that was in Him. Jesus took *every* sickness, disease, and "condition" on his body so that we would not have to bear it. He gave us authority over all of that. He took the horrific beating on His body that satisfied the demand of us having to "live with" any form of being unhealthy (1 Peter 2:24). The Bible emphatically states that He has *surely* borne our sicknesses so we can be well. (Matthew 8:17).

Communion, taken in faith and not as a ritual, reminds us to see our sickness on His body, not ours. Taken often, communion reinforces the truth of His body bearing everything that comes to attack our bodies. This is why Jesus repeatedly said in John 6 that He was the Bread from

Heaven, knowing that His body would be broken so that ours would be whole.

He greatly desires that we live an abundant life—one without sickness, lack, fear, or condemnation. Having children is a part of the abundant life He has planned for us. He desires that we would have children and teach them of His love for them. He knows that every person who accepts Him as Savior will be a part of His eternal family.

Jesus gave Himself so we would not only go to heaven when we die but to also give us an abundant life here on earth, exchanging our weaknesses, infirmities, and shortcomings for His strengths, divine health and overflowing supply. Taking communion is a reminder of this great exchange that He made possible.

Speak the Word: I take communion often to remember the covenant I have with God, which was established because of his love for me, through the body and blood of Jesus.

More Encouragement: Luke 22:19,20; Colossians 1:14, 20-22

Dig Deeper: When you take communion, how do you remind yourself of the Father's love for you and of Jesus' finished work on the cross for the healing of your body?

Confidence in Action #5

Take communion regularly and frequently at your home.

Receive God's forgiveness and grace so that you can enjoy living the abundant life He has planned for you. It's time to get rid of anything that makes you pull away from God. It's not just your time and activities that can distract you. Emotions like bitterness and unforgiveness can make you withdraw from Him.

Remember, your faith works by love (Galatians 5:6) so as you receive communion, be ever conscious of *God's love for you*. Jesus died so that you can live in His righteousness knowing that you have been made a worthy recipient of the Father's unconditional love, kindness, grace, and goodness.

Reflections

Are You Angry with God?

*"And I will make an everlasting covenant with them,
promising not to stop doing good for them. I will put a
desire in their hearts to worship me, and they will never
leave Me."*
~ Jeremiah 32:40 (NLT) ~

I t's natural to feel angry with God when you desperately want to get pregnant, you're praying to get pregnant, and still nothing happens.

It's natural to think He's not hearing you. It's natural to think He doesn't care about your situation or that He has forgotten you. It's natural to wonder if God is angry with you for what you've done (or haven't done) and if infertility might be your punishment.

Yes, those are all perfectly natural thoughts and almost everyone you know probably supports you in those thoughts. BUT GOD DOES NOT CALL BELIEVERS IN JESUS TO THINK *NATURAL* THOUGHTS! He calls us to think *above* natural thoughts. He calls us to think *hope-filled* thoughts. He calls us to think His SUPERNATURAL thoughts (Philippians 4:8).

He wants us to remember how great His love is for us through Jesus. God has given us the ability and power to cast down and reject thoughts and imaginations that are not of Him (2 Corinthians 10:5). Those thoughts and imaginations would include being angry with God.

The best way to combat any anger you may be feeling towards God is to concentrate more on how He showed His great love for you through Jesus. Concentrate and think thoughts about how God loves you so much and only wants the best for you. Think about how God greatly values you to the point that He was willing to give His only beloved Son to suffer a death that should have been yours. Think about how special you must be to Jesus that He would do that on your behalf.

There's a bonus too—when you receive Jesus' love, it also blesses you in your body! Infertility is not stronger than Jesus' unconditional love for you. The more you think about, hear about, and talk about His love, the more it will diminish and eliminate the anger you may experience.

Jesus desires a loving relationship with you because you were born with a destiny and purpose that can be achieved only through a life with Him. Breakthrough comes when you experience that intimate love of Jesus. He loves you with an everlasting love (Jeremiah 31:3; John 15:9). He desires that you look to Him and trust Him in overcoming every battle, every angry thought, and every tough situation—even infertility.

As for the thought that infertility may be your punishment, it is _not_. Jesus satisfied any and all punishments required for your disobedience, your promiscuity, your neglect, everything! God does not remember any of those things. He has chosen to forget them (Psalm 103:12; Hebrews 10:14-17). Be thankful He loves you so much that He has wiped your slate clean with His blood! Because of Jesus, you are no longer under condemnation and are now qualified to enjoy His goodness, His grace, and His provision (Romans 8:1).

114

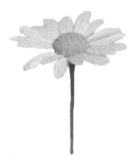

Speak the Word: I am valued and loved by God. He only wants to do good for me. I bring my emotions and thoughts into captivity to concentrate on His love for me.

More Encouragement: Hebrews 10:4,5; John 17:23

Dig Deeper: How can you best process any anger that you may have towards God? What Scripture verses would be helpful in assuring you of God's love for you?

God's Love for You

"Yes, I have loved you with an everlasting love; Therefore with lovingkindness I have drawn you." ~ Jeremiah 31:3 ~

Love is always the motivator behind Jesus' actions. His love is always available for us to take hold of and bask in. He always wants the best for us and He deeply desires to bring us out of dark, dire circumstances. Jesus has provided His love and power for us to use in our lives to break off the yokes and chokers that were put on us by the devil.

Infertility is a shadow of death and is like a choker on your reproductive system, preventing it from bringing forth life. Through the sacrifice of Jesus, that choker was utterly destroyed. Psalm 107:14 says, "He brought them out of darkness and the shadow of death, and breaks their bands asunder."

When I was a teen in the 1970's, choker necklaces were in style. They were typically made out of a strip of leather or ribbon that had to be tied around your neck. If tied too tightly, they felt as if someone's hand was around your neck, squeezing and literally choking you and keeping you from taking a breath.

That's what infertility felt like to me—as if I was being prevented from doing the very basic thing that allows the human life cycle to continue. I would sometimes think, "Having a baby should be easy, after all, how many teenaged girls are becoming pregnant the very *first* time

116

they have sex?" It wasn't easy for us, and it felt like we were being held captive in the "Land of Infertility". Why couldn't I click my heels together like Dorothy in the Wizard of Oz and leave that alien, hostile place called Infertility? I wanted to be released from those infertility chokers and move on to the "Land of Pregnancy"!

Are you reading this and nodding your head because you too feel like you are being held captive? Well, God is always working to set people free! He wants to set women free from the choke hold of infertility. Keep looking to Jesus. Believe in His love and His mighty power.

If you lack confidence in God's love for you and need assurance that He wants you free, ask Him for a deeper revelation and a clearer view of His love. He will surely give it to you. Pray the Word from Ephesians 3:17-18, "I am rooted and grounded in God's love because Jesus lives in me. By faith, I comprehend with all saints, every dimension of His unconditional love for me."

Speak the Word: God's love for me is powerful, unconditional, and everlasting!

More Encouragement: 1 Timothy 1:14

Dig Deeper: What have you found to be the most effective way to focus on God's love for you?

Built to be Tough

*"You therefore must endure hardship as a good soldier of
Jesus Christ."*
~ 2 Timothy 2:3 ~

If you are a believer in Jesus Christ, you are without
question built to be tough against the enemy, the devil.
You already have the capability built into your newly
created spirit to withstand difficult circumstances. That
capability is called HOPE. You have that capability
because you were made to be like Jesus and Jesus *always*
has a hopeful view of life.

Choose to see life from His hope-filled perspective. Do you
think He looks at infertility and cringes, running away in
fear, or that He loses hope that the condition can't be
changed? NO! He looks at it though eyes of hope with
anticipation that it will be changed because He has already
overcome it through His death and resurrection. He's just
waiting on you and me to use His power that He's given us
to manifest the change so we can physically see it. Jesus
has sent His Holy Spirit to live in us and to empower us
(Acts 1:8). That's how we can confidently expect to live
each day as a day meant for taking territory for His
kingdom and establishing His covenant.

Our door of hope, our entrance into His state of confident
expectation, is worship. The Bible says that he who dwells
in the secret place of the Most High shall abide (live) in His
shadow (Psalm 91:1). Since the God of the universe casts a
rather broad shadow, it is safe to say there's room for

everyone who wants to be there. We get there and remain there by seeking Him, by communicating with Him. It's how we avoid hopelessness.

It can sometimes be easy to get into a state of hopelessness. When you dwell on a negative sad thought long enough, you begin to believe it as truth and that makes it hard to find reason to hope. But biblical hope does not disappoint (Romans 5:5). You avoid hopelessness when you make a decision to think the way God thinks about infertility---He doesn't support it nor does He cause it. When you choose to have hope and think about yourself the way God thinks about you, it raises your hope and helps you see a bright future. It enables you to be tough and to endure. See yourself filled with hope, living in God's grace, knowing you are special to Him. See yourself in the midst of a happy family, playing with your children, and enjoying life.

See yourself starting each day anticipating God's goodness. Start TODAY!

Speak the Word: I endure the trials of life knowing that as I stand on the firm foundation of the Word, God causes me to triumph in Christ.

More Encouragement: 1 Corinthians 15:57; John 16:33; Ephesians 6:13

Dig Deeper: What will you do to open the door of hope each morning so that you set a positive tone for your day?

Ask For a Child of Promise

"Now we, brethren, as Isaac was, are the children of promise." ~ Galatians 4:28 ~

After trying for many months to get pregnant, I realized that I was trying to *force* it to happen. As a result, the stress and disappointment started to mount.

I had grown up in a home where there was love but also a good deal of stress, usually about financial issues. My parents loved me and loved the Lord, but just didn't know how to handle the stress very well. I did not want my home environment and marriage relationship to go down that same path.

I had to make a choice. I could continue to try everything to make it happen myself and get stressed out more and more as each monthly cycle came and went, *or*, I could trust God and be patient for His promise to manifest in my life.

The Bible tells the account of how Sarah and Abraham had reached the ages of 80+ and were still childless, which meant no biological heir to their household (Genesis 16 and 17). Sarah, in her desperation, encouraged Abraham to have sex with someone else to produce a child. Sarah and Abraham decided to "make this thing happen" by having a baby through a surrogate, Hagar, their Egyptian slave. Hagar gave birth to a son, Ishmael, when Abraham was 86 years old. But was this child the fulfillment of what God had promised in the covenant He had made with Abraham? (Genesis 15:1-6, 18)

Apparently not! God corrected them, letting them know that their covenant posterity was not through Ishmael but through a son yet to be born that they were to name Isaac. Sarah got ahead of God in trying to do everything in her power to have a child. **But God had a *better* plan.** The child that He had promised would indeed come through her body, even though she was "ninety-something", far from today's usual childbearing age of "twenty-something". When Sarah heard from God for herself and trusted Him by allowing His plan to become her plan, she got pregnant. She gave birth to Isaac, a child of promise, just as God had declared in His conversation with Abraham a year earlier (Genesis 17:16-21).

I decided the best thing was for me to want a "child of promise", an Isaac, not an Ishmael. I wanted the child God intended for us to have through His grace, not the one I would make happen through any means necessary. This decision made it so much easier to walk away from the prospect of many months of infertility treatments and the burdensome expense of those procedures.

My prayer for a child changed. Instead of "God please, please, please let me have a baby!" and "God, why isn't it my turn yet?" or "Please let me get pregnant next month!" I began to pray "Lord, give me an Isaac, not an Ishmael." I only wanted a child of promise.

God answered that prayer. Our son has been a blessing since God first formed him in my womb. Each time we decided to have another child, before becoming pregnant, I asked God for an Isaac, not an Ishmael—I wanted a child of promise, a child who would lead a blessed life and who would bless others. Twice more, God answered that prayer. Our younger son and our daughter have also been blessings from the time God formed them in my womb. Each of our children is blessed to be a blessing! Nothing could stop His plan once I began to rest in Him and allow His plan to become my plan.

Speak the Word: I do not allow my heart to be troubled. Instead I trust and believe in Jesus' plan for me and I receive His peace.

More Encouragement: John 14:1, 27; Matthew 11:28, 29

Dig Deeper: During this season of infertility, how have your prayers changed? What additional adjustments should you make to the way that you pray?

Don't Give Up!

"Be strong in the Lord, and in His mighty power. Use every piece of God's armor to resist the enemy in the time of evil, so that after the battle you will still be standing firm."
~ Ephesians 6:10, 13 (NLT) ~

It's easy to give up when your enemy looms large over you, or when you've been fighting for so long it looks like there will be no end to the battle.

Imagine you are a soldier in a war, fighting for your life and the lives of your fellow soldiers. You're armed with many powerful weapons—grenades, automatic guns, and knives hidden in various parts of your clothing and gear. When you've been fighting for 18 hours non-stop, having to dodge bullets and explosions all around you, you're sure to be physically tired, emotionally drained, and ready to quit. But you can't give up because just 10 feet away from you is your buddy who you must protect.

The battle against infertility is much the same. You're involved in a fight that continues 24/7--- it never stops. It's a mental and spiritual battle. You're equipped with many weapons—truth, righteousness, peace, and faith—all very powerful. But after many months and maybe even years of fighting, you find yourself growing battle-weary. In the midst of that weariness, God says "Persevere! Don't give up, continue to stand!" You may not know how close you are to breakthrough and ultimate victory over infertility, but He does.

The Bible tells us of many battles that David fought. His most famous was against the giant enemy Goliath. His odds for winning the fight were extremely low when you account for his lack of training, weapons and armor. But David had declared that He was in the army of the Lord, God Almighty, and therefore he stood firm, confident that God was his refuge and his fortress.

A refuge is a place of safety and rest, where there's no anxiety. A fortress is an impenetrable place from which to fight. David trusted that in God he was safe, and he rested in the fact that he would be victorious in the fight because God was on his side. Even when no one else believed in his impending victory, David put on *God's* armor and went out to fight for the men, women and children of his nation. He trusted God and did not give up when faced with a gigantic enemy and seemingly impossible odds. David won the battle. He defeated his enemy, all because he trusted God.

You may feel like you're facing a gigantic enemy and impossible odds to overcome infertility. Instead of giving up in despair, encourage yourself and declare like David did, "God is my refuge and fortress; I trust Him" (Psalm 91:2). Know that you are safe in Him. Know that when you fight from God's vantage point while using His weapons and believing that you have victory in Him, this enemy *will* retreat in defeat.

Thank God for victory NOW!

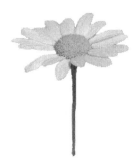

Speak the Word: When I am challenged, I stand firm and encourage myself, for God is my refuge and fortress. I trust Him and I trust in His Word. I thank God for my victory!

More Encouragement: 2 Timothy 2:3; Micah 3:8; Psalm 91

Dig Deeper: In what ways do you use "every piece of God's armor" as Paul described in Ephesians 6:10-18? Do you *expect* to be standing in victory?

Stir It Up!

"Rejoice in the Lord always. Again I will say, rejoice!"
~ Philippians 4:4 ~

Keep up your guard to keep depression from setting in when you've been diagnosed with having infertility "issues". One bad thought may come, like, "we may never have kids" and then you think about it over and over and over again. Dwelling on that thought and the other discouraging thoughts that are sure to come along with it can put you on the path to the dark ditch of depression.

So how do you avoid it? You have to stir up the joy inside you! Joy is bigger than your emotions. Joy does not depend on how you feel. Experiencing joy depends on your will. It requires that you make a decision to rejoice even when you don't feel like it. It requires that you choose to replace the discouraging hopeless thoughts with thoughts that are lovely, of good report, and that are true, which means they are based on the Word of God (Philippians 4:8).

There are a variety of ways to stir up the joy within you. Begin by being thankful for the basics like life itself. Thank God for His Word working in your life and for the blood and body of Jesus that forgives, saves, and heals you. Connect with God through prayer and meditating on His Word, always praising Him for His goodness. Listen to uplifting music that reminds you of how God loves you. Stir up joy by singing and dancing. The Bible tells us that in His presence is the *fullness* of joy. So enter His presence with thanksgiving. Give Him thanks for His love and His grace working in your life.

You will become stronger with the might of God as you choose to rejoice and connect with God because the joy of the Lord is your strength (Nehemiah 8:10). Joy will put you in a strong place, His secret place, so that every chain the devil has tried to throw on you to keep you in bondage to depressing thoughts will be destroyed.

Make a decision today to stir up your joy!

Speak the Word: I *choose* to be joyful today. I choose to dwell in God's presence because it is there that I experience fullness of joy.

More Encouragement: Psalm 5:11; Psalm 16:11

Dig Deeper: What would stir up a greater sense of joy in your life?

Be Specific About What You Ask For

"When you pray, don't babble on and on as people of other religions do. They think their prayers are answered only by repeating their words again and again.
~ Matthew 6:7 (NLT) ~

It's important when you pray to ask God specifically for what you desire and then stand on His Word and watch Him work. When you're specific in asking for something, you have it clear in your mind what to expect.

You may want to begin to think about the kind of experience you want to have once you become pregnant and then, ask God for it. After seeing my best friend have a very hard time with morning sickness, I specifically asked God to allow me to have a pregnancy without morning sickness. I had no symptoms of morning sickness. You see, you don't *have to* experience things the way everyone else does.

Maybe you want to have a pregnancy without excessive weight gain, especially if you already experience health issues from being overweight. If you are currently overweight, why not do yourself and your baby a favor? Make a decision, purpose in your heart, be determined to lose a specific amount of weight in a specific amount of time for the health of your baby and then take action to make it happen. This may feel like a sacrifice on your part, but trust me; it will NOT be the last time you make a sacrifice for your child. Just consider this practice for all the times of sacrifice that lay ahead.

Find scriptures that encourage you on whatever you're specifically asking God for. Take his promises to heart as if He was speaking them directly to you (because He is) and then stand on them---believe they will come to pass. Persevere in speaking those promises so you can get your faith established in them by hearing them (Romans 10:17).

Whatever you ask God for, be specific, find His promise about it, and then think about that promise, speak it, believe it, and expect it. Joshua 1:8 says, "to do these things daily"—in other words, consistently. Consistency is key when dealing with the things of God. Isaiah 55:11 tells us the benefit of consistency in the Word—God's Word will not return to him void (it will not be useless or of no effect), but it will accomplish what He sent it to do in your life.

This should give you confidence that the vision you have for your child is not empty or without effect when you connect that vision to, and bathe it in, the great anointing of the Word of God.

Speak the Word: I am specific in what I ask of God by finding what I desire in His Word, speaking and believing that because of God's grace, it shall come to pass.

More Encouragement: Matthew 7:7, 8; Hebrews 3:14

Dig Deeper: Find a scripture that relates to having a child (find many in the Appendix). Write it down. Consistently pray it aloud, giving thanks in advance (Philippians 4:6).

Rest

*"If we believe, though, we'll experience that state of
resting. But not if we don't have faith."*
~ *Hebrews 4:3 (MSG)* ~

Infertility can be such a driving force and such a heavy
burden.

It can cause you to become hardened and turn away from
the very one who has made the way for you to be rescued
from it!

God's Word tells us that *in Christ*, we can experience rest.
This is not speaking of the physical type of rest but rather
the relief, ease, and refreshing of your mind and emotions.
His rest brings a comfortable, blessed quietness into your
life (Matthew 11:28-29). How do you enter into His rest?

The Bible tells us in Hebrews 3 and 4 that entering into
God's rest is tied to having faith in Jesus and becoming
more intimately acquainted with Him so that trusting Him
becomes effortless. It is found by spending time in His
presence, cultivating a relationship with Him. We are
encouraged to hold on to our confidence in Him, being firm
and unshaken in our trust in God and what He has spoken
about our situation. We are encouraged to take advantage
of His offer to rest and be without anxiety in Him and to do
it TODAY.

The Israelites, who refused to be persuaded by God's words
while in the wilderness with Moses, were not able to enter

into His rest. They chose to be anxious and look elsewhere for answers to their problems. Their unbelief shut them out (Hebrews 11:19; Numbers 14:1-35).

We're blessed that through Jesus, God's promise of rest is still offered to you and me today. By having absolute trust and confidence in the wisdom that He's spoken, in His love for us, in His dominion over all other powers, we can be secure in His rest.

All the anxiety about infertility you felt as soon as you woke up this morning was not sent from God. All the anxiety you may sometimes feel even as you and your husband are having sexual intercourse—as you wonder if this will be another failed attempt at conceiving a baby— was not sent from God. God repeatedly offers His rest to you, everyday. Trust in His unfailing love, His powerful words, and the completed work of deliverance through Jesus on your behalf.

Jesus Himself said, *"Come to me all you who labor and are heavy-laden and overburdened and I will cause you to rest. I will ease and relieve and refresh your souls."* (Matthew 11:28 AMP)

See Jesus with open arms, waiting for you to accept His invitation to come to Him, so that you can flow with Him in the fullness of God's grace, experiencing His peaceful rest and His guaranteed victory. Your rest and your breakthrough are in His presence because Jesus has already done *everything* necessary for your victory. Choose to focus on and rest in the love and the FINISHED work of Jesus.

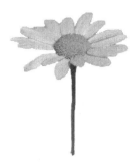

Speak the Word: I have faith in the promises of God. I believe they are true for me. In His presence there is great grace, peace, and rest. I enter into His rest because Jesus has already done *everything* necessary for my victory.

More Encouragement: Psalm 16:8, 9; Hebrews 4:9-11; Acts 2:26

Dig Deeper: In the past, when have you experienced breakthrough by resting in Jesus' love and provision? How can you do so now?

The Fight

"No, despite all these things, overwhelming victory is ours through Christ, who loved us."
~ Romans 8:37 (NLT) ~

Do you consider yourself a warrior? Have you ever put up a fight for anything that you intensely desired? Well, that's what it's going to take to overcome in this battle against infertility. But the battle is not against infertility itself. Jesus has already conquered that in His death and resurrection and made you an heir of His victory. Your battle is actually against the thoughts that bombard your mind and cause you to doubt the victory that Jesus won on your behalf. It's the fight to *keep* the faith!

I had a tough time with what I call "stinkin' thinkin'". Thoughts like "She doesn't even take good care of the child she has. Why does she have one and I don't?" or, "Wait a minute! She didn't even *want* a baby and *she's* pregnant?" All those thoughts are intended to keep you distracted so you won't think about the goodness of God, or His power to turn your situation around.

Your fight is taking place between your ears---in your thought-life. But Zechariah 10:5 encourages us stating, "They shall fight because the Lord is with them." Even though you don't see Him, even though your pregnancy may be taking WAY too long to manifest itself, you must hang on to the truth that God is indeed with you in the fight. Romans 8:31 assures us that "if God is for us, who can be against us?" In other words, God is on your side so nobody can defeat you when you acknowledge that He's the "big dog" on your team and He's already won the battle against the enemy.

You have the privilege to tag team with Jesus in this fight so you can enjoy victory even though you didn't have to fight the battle directly with the enemy. Jesus already fought and won the title of Lord of All. Therefore, *you* are the victor, *you* are the overcomer, and *you* are the conqueror because of His victory.

Speak the Word: Overwhelming victory is mine because of Jesus' victory over the enemy and because of His love for me.

More Encouragement: Romans 8:31-39; 1 Timothy 6:12; 2 Timothy 4:7

Dig Deeper: In what area of your life do you find the fight against stinkin' thinkin' to be the toughest? Why?

Let the Word
Do Its Work

"The LORD said to me, "You have seen correctly, for I am watching to see that my word is fulfilled."
~ Jeremiah 1:12 (NIV) ~

D o you believe in the integrity of God's Word, the Bible? Do you regard the Word as being uncorrupted and perfect?

Is it reliable in its instruction to you and how it relates to your life? Do you believe that it provides wisdom for everything you need for living a good life (2Peter 1:3-4)?

The integrity of God's Word is something you can count on. Depend on what God has said as a personal letter of promise to you and treat it as the final authority when you're searching for solutions to life's problems. Value the Word as your lifesaver and life-giver.

In order to use the Word to overcome infertility, receive the Word as the absolute, undeniable, unchanging truth. Believe what it says. Do what it says. When you believe it in your heart (not just in your head), you're enabled to possess the blessing inside of you and change your circumstances on the outside of you.

There's no weakness in the effectiveness of the Word. It *can* change this circumstance of infertility. Rest assured

135

that what God has said does not change simply because He's tired that day, or because someone else ticked Him off earlier in the day, or because you said or did something to disappoint Him.

Trust in God's gift of grace that He imparted to you through Jesus and allow the power of His grace to work in you and for you. You allow it to work by resting in His love and His victory over infertility. His grace is always turned "on". So because it NEVER gets turned "off", you can trust that what He has promised is forever settled and will not change (Psalm 119:89).

God hasn't, doesn't, and will not change (Malachi 3:6; Hebrews 13:8). God is not two-faced. He will not "flip-flop" on what He has promised to you. If you find that He has promised it in His Word, you can certainly count on it.

God said that whoever seeks Him would find Him. Search His Word and find His promises that you can stand on against infertility. His Word will become a reality to you. It must become more real to you than the problem of infertility.

Have faith in it and receive it as a personal word from Jesus about victory over infertility through Him. Allow that word to be magnified and loom larger than your circumstances. Choose to believe His Word no matter your circumstances and let the Word do its work.

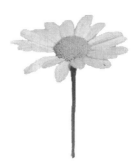

Speak the Word: I believe that as I speak God's Word in faith, He is watching over His Word to fulfill it.

More Encouragement: 2 Corinthians 1:20 and 4:7-10,13; James 1:17

Dig Deeper: What do you see when you envision the fertility promises in God's Word being fulfilled in your life? Write it down and review it often (Habakkuk 2:2).

Weary of Others?

*"But those who hope in the Lord will renew their strength.
They will soar on wings like eagles; they will run and not
grow weary, they will walk and not be faint."*
~ *Isaiah 40:31 (NIV)* ~

If you've shared the doctor's report of infertility with
family and friends you may have grown weary of their
suggestions, advice, and anecdotes.

You may have been told to try some "natural remedies" or
even superstitious practices. The good news is you can turn
to one source of healing that you'll never get tired of
hearing—the Word of God.

There are many wives tales about why women don't get
pregnant and probably even more tales about how a woman
can increase her chances of getting pregnant. I'd rather not
gamble and take "chances". I'd much rather rely on a sure
thing—God's truth. Truth is absolute and can be counted as
reliable.

Proverbs 4:20-22 says: *"My son, give attention to my
words; Incline your ear to my sayings. Do not let them
depart from your eyes; Keep them in the midst of your
heart; For they are life to those who find them, And health
to all their flesh."* In other words, God's Word is medicine.
You don't have to pay for it, you can't overdose on it, and
it is available worldwide and at any time of the day or
night! That scripture says His Word is also *life* to those that
find it.

So seek for it as if you're on a treasure hunt because it is indeed a valuable treasure. When others may be speaking doom and gloom, look for promises in the Word that speak life to your spirit, soul, and body. An example of an encouraging scripture is Genesis 30:22-23 (AMP): *"Then God remembered Rachel and answered her pleading and made it possible for her to have children. And [now for the first time] she became pregnant and bore a son."*

Earlier in that passage, we see Rachel as a woman who had not fully trusted God to come through in blessing her with a child. Despite this, God was faithful and gave her a son, whom she named Joseph. He would grow to become a victor over many trials and be given the second highest position in all the land of Egypt, saving the Israelites from certain devastation during a great famine in the land.

Another example is found in Psalm 139:13 (NLT): *"You made all the delicate, inner parts of my body and knit me together in my mother's womb."* It goes on to say in the next verse that God is the Creator of all things and we are fearfully and wonderfully made. God plants life in our womb, which starts at conception, and His intention is for parents to raise that baby to be a blessing to its family and to the world.

It's understandable if you're weary of hearing other people tell you what to do to change the circumstances of infertility. But always, always rejoice in the remedy that God offers, for His truth CAN change your circumstances.

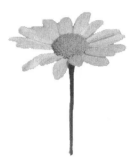

Speak the Word: My hope is in God and I do not grow weary. His truth strengthens me to persevere.

More Encouragement: Galatians 6:9; 2 Thessalonians 3:13

Dig Deeper: What is it that spurs you on to persevere?

Confidence in Action

#6

Consistently speak God's Word without fear and doubt. Know that God loves YOU. He loves you so much that He gave up His only child, His sinless son Jesus, to be used as the perfect substitute and sacrifice for you. It was the only thing He could do to make you righteous and thus restore you as a part of His family. You see, family is of the utmost importance to God. So trust Him to help you to start, build and raise your family.

Reflections

Declare the End

"Declaring the end from the beginning, and from ancient times things that are not yet done, saying, 'My counsel shall stand, and I will do all My pleasure.'"
~ Isaiah 46:10 ~

God declares the end of a thing at its beginning. So do as God does—speak the end result that you desire to see.

Find in the Bible what He has already spoken about your situation. Then, as you pray about it, include speaking that Word in your prayer. The Bible says, "He sent His Word and healed them and delivered them from their destructions" (Psalm 107:20).

The Word is the way of escape from things that come to destroy wholeness in your body, mind, spirit, finances, and relationships. Infertility is definitely one of the destructions that God delivers us from. I'm living proof!

Whether you are praying for yourself, a family member, or a friend, praying the Word of God works! Joshua 1:8, Psalm 119:13 and Proverbs 22:18 all encourage believers to read and speak the Word of God repeatedly. Why? The answer is contained in Isaiah 55:11—His Word does not return to Him void. His Word returns to Him by us speaking it and those words will not fall to the ground without effect; they will produce the purpose and results for which He spoke them.

When thoughts of fear and doubt about overcoming childlessness arise, speak the Word—say what God has said about your situation. Speak with faith, expectancy and gratefulness. This helps you to focus on God and not on the problem. He's bigger and more powerful than any problem you may be facing. He gladly and lovingly responds to your faith in His Word. See your desired end in the Word and continually speak that Word until you see it in your life.

Speak the Word: I am an imitator of God. I declare my desired end from the beginning, relying on God's Word to make it so.

More Encouragement: 2 Corinthians 4:13,18

Dig Deeper: In what scriptures do you see your desired end result? How consistently declaring them?

Seedtime and Harvest

"While the earth remains, seedtime and harvest, cold and heat, winter and summer, and day and night shall not cease." ~ Genesis 8:22 ~

God has declared that the principle of sowing seed and reaping a harvest is His way of doing things and it will not cease. In explaining the parable of the sower, Jesus said that the seed represents the Word of God (Luke 8:11). The Word of God, when planted in the good soil of our believing heart, will always produce a good harvest. Likewise, every word that we speak is a seed sown that will produce a harvest, whether good or bad.

What are you saying about having children? What "seeds" are you sowing through the words that you speak? Are you saying things in your everyday conversations that will produce weeds of infertility in your life or will a fruitful crop be produced by your words? A fruitful crop cannot and will not come from a barren field where nothing has been sown.

Any farmer knows that every seed, in due season, produces after its own kind. A potato seed produces potatoes; an orange seed produces a tree of oranges, and so on. Likewise, your words act as seeds and your words of worry and fear of infertility produce after their kind, prolonging and even strengthening infertility's grip. But, if you're speaking words of faith about God and His love for you, words of expectancy and hope, words of thankfulness, then you are planting seeds that will loose the grip of infertility and will produce a fruitful harvest.

There is a spirit of life or a spirit of death in *everything* that we say (Proverbs 18:21). Our words show what our faith is in at that very moment. Satan's only hope is that you are planting bad seed for your future with the words that come from your mouth. Your life today is the harvest of what you've spoken in the yesterdays of your life. I challenge you to purposely listen to yourself more closely each day in your normal "everyday" conversation and determine if you are speaking life or death about overcoming infertility. If you find yourself saying things to friends, co-workers and family that do not line up with what God says, change your words!

By changing your words and speaking what Jesus said, you are changing your harvest to one of life. Jesus said that His words are spirit, life, and truth (John 6:63). Saying what He said brings life to our circumstances. Saying what He said produces a bountiful and fruitful crop, not an infertile, barren one.

"Life" is the harvest of the Word of God. What harvest do you desire to see in your life? What are you speaking *today* that will develop and shape the 'todays' of your future?

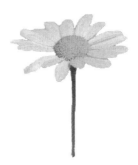

> **Speak the Word:** I sow good seed with the words of my mouth by speaking the Word of God and I expect a harvest of "life".
>
> **More Encouragement:** Matthew 12:35-37; Proverbs 12:14
>
> **Dig Deeper:** What changes could you make so your daily conversations align with what God has said in His Word, especially in His promises of fertility?

Refuse Hopelessness

"Be of good courage, And He shall strengthen your heart,
all you who hope in the LORD."
~ Psalm 31:24 ~

No matter how long you've been facing the problem of infertility, you can still have hope because your resources or your negative circumstances do not limit God. He can only be limited by your unbelief in His willingness to do something on your behalf (Psalm 78:41). Your hope must be based on the unbreakable covenant promises that God has established to bring unlimited possibilities to you.

Mark 9:23 states that "all things are possible to him (her) who believes." So refuse to allow hopelessness to settle into your life. Instead, let hope take root and grow in every area of your life, especially regarding getting pregnant and having a healthy baby. You may not always clearly see God doing something in your life's circumstances but that does not mean that He's not listening to your prayers. Nor does it mean that He does not care about what's happening in your life. Sometimes, God is working things out in the background because he knows that our faith needs to be put into action in order for it to grow. No matter what, you can rest assured that He is on your side, working things out for your good.

Seek God through prayers that are based on His promises of provision, not prayers that are only based on need and worry. Provision-based prayers are faith-based prayers. They acknowledge that Jesus has already done what's necessary to provide for your need. We are assured in 2 Peter 1:3 that God has already given us everything we need in life, through faith in Jesus. As you trust in that promise of abundant provision you will receive it. Have confidence in His wisdom and power. Have confidence in His love for you.

Give no authority to any amount of hopelessness you're currently experiencing in your life. Become promise-minded and God's-answer-minded. *That's how you'll keep hope alive.*

Speak the Word: I keep my hope alive in Christ Jesus by believing that He *is* the answer for every need that I have.

More Encouragement: Psalm 16:9; Psalm 38:15; Jeremiah 17:7

Dig Deeper: What are your prayers based upon…fear or God's promises?

Envisioning the Promise

"And God said, 'Let there be light': and there was light."
~ Genesis 1:3 ~

God called forth light in the midst of total darkness. He did not bemoan the fact that the darkness existed.

He did not fear that He couldn't see the end of it. Instead, He spoke what He wanted to see and He called forth light. You are made in His image so, by faith, you should do the same. Infertility is a source of darkness in your life but God brings His light to your circumstances and the light chases the darkness away. In the midst of the "darkness" of infertility, choose to call forth the "light" of a fertile, healthy womb, trusting in the grace and favor of Jesus.

Jesus said that when we are united to Him and allow His Words to become vital to our lives, they become a way of life and a way *to* life. We can ask what we want according to His Word and it will be done. Have confidence that He hears and answers your prayers that are based on faith in His Word.

In 1 Kings 18:41-46, there is an account of the prophet Elijah envisioning the promise God had made. He began to *expect* that what God had said would manifest. In this account, we see him speaking the God-given vision and calling it forth. Elijah made a declaration of God's promise of rain —"There is the sound of abundance of rain." He said this even before he physically saw any clouds or heard any sound in the air. He envisioned the rain, though he had no present physical evidence that it would happen.

Elijah was operating on what God had already said. His faith sustained him as he anticipated the rain without any evidence that it was forthcoming. His words aligned with God's words as he sent his servant to look for clouds over the sea. Seven times the servant went to look for evidence and found none. But finally he returned to Elijah with a report that he could see a little cloud, the size of a man's hand rising from the sea. From that seemingly insignificant bit of evidence, Elijah shouted to his servant, "Hurry! Climb into your chariot and go – if you don't the rain will stop you."

He expected the rain simply because God had said it would happen (1 Kings 18:1). Elijah didn't know how or when it would happen but he had confidence that God's Word was *his* truth. A torrential rainstorm came as a result of Elijah's **expectation** of God to follow through on what He had said.

Spend time envisioning what you desire. Visualize yourself being pregnant and it will begin to expand your hope! Start seeing yourself holding your baby using your "eyes of faith". See yourself cuddling your baby, singing to and feeding him/her, taking the baby for walks, etc. Then, speak the vision that you see and call it forth in faith, in Jesus' name.

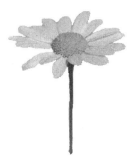

Speak the Word: I trust in the grace of God and call forth the light of a healthy fertile womb.

More Encouragement: John 15:7, 16

Dig Deeper: What promises has God already fulfilled in other areas of your life? Use those fulfillments to bring light and hope to this fertility struggle.

Praise Him

"The LORD is my strength, my shield from every danger. I trust in him with all my heart. He helps me, and my heart is filled with joy. I burst out in songs of thanksgiving."
~ Psalm 28:7 (NLT) ~

Each day, take a moment to praise God. Sing a song to Him—it will improve your mood, increase your joy, and generate strength within you.

Sing a song of thanks. Tell Him how grateful you are for all He's done, is doing and will do on your behalf.

Sing a love song to Him. Let God know that you accept His love for you. Tell Him how you love Him.

Sing a song of worship. Acknowledge that he alone is God and that there is no one else like Him. Adore Him simply because of who he is.

In Isaiah 54:1, God specifically encourages the infertile (barren) woman to praise Him:

> "Sing, those of you married women who are infertile. Sing and shout those of you who have not given birth to a child. Praise Him so that the number of the children of the married wives will outnumber those of single women." (*Paraphrased*)

Praise is the powerful place in which God dwells (Psalm 22:3) and manifests Himself as strong. It's in that place where things change because of His presence. So sing a new song to Him. Allow God to put a song in your heart and then sing it back to Him. Singing praise to Him is like putting on a brand new, fashionable outfit. It puts some pep in your step. It makes you feel lighter inside. It makes you feel better about yourself and life in general. Choose right now to take off that heavy, burdensome garment of shame along with the depressing thoughts that it causes, and put on God's light and airy, joy-giving garment of praise.

Speak the Word: The Lord is my Strength and my Shield. With my song I will praise Him!

More Encouragement: Psalm 89:15,16; Psalm 27:6; Psalm 109:30

Dig Deeper: How quickly do you deal with depressing thoughts when they come? What strategies can you use against them so that you avoid a downward emotional spiral?

Preparation

"If only you would prepare your heart and lift up your hands to him in prayer!
~ Job 11:13 (NLT) ~

Before we got to the point of deciding we were ready to have children, my husband and I were pretty arrogant about the kind of parents we would be. You know what I mean, looking at people with a screaming, fussy toddler and shaking our heads, commenting that we'd never allow our child to behave that way. We thought we'd be "super parents"; knowing exactly what to do in every situation so that our children would always be obedient, cooperative, clean from head to toe, polite, etc. We thought parenthood would be easy for us!

We quickly learned from babysitting our very young godchildren that our way of thinking was naïve. Our lack of experience in dealing with a very young human being was quite evident on the first night we babysat. It was a reality check—one that we really needed. Their parents actually became excellent examples for us as we continued to "watch" them raise their children even through the teenage years.

Finding scriptures on parenting and meditating on them became a priority for me. I knew that if we were going to raise godly, happy children, we would need God's help. We would also need the encouragement and wise counsel of friends and family in order to set an atmosphere of joy, peace, and love in our home. All of this was in preparation for the children with which we believed God would bless us even though we were still childless at the time.

Some scriptures I repeatedly read, prayed, and confessed were:
- Deuteronomy 11:18-19
- Deuteronomy 6:6-9
- Proverbs 22:6
- Proverbs 15:1
- Ephesians 6:4
- Proverbs 5:18
- 1 Timothy 2:15
- John 16:21

I hope you'll use these scriptures and find others, as God directs you, to pray for the children you desire to have. This will begin to set the atmosphere in your home and prepare you and your husband as parents. Open yourself to how God would have you to pray His Word and believe in the promises contained in His Word.

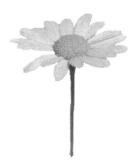

A Prayer: Lord, I pray these promises and instructions from you will be a comfort to us, that they will be fulfilled in the children we are to have and also in us as parents. Through faith, I believe Your Word for my family, and receive all the blessings that follow. In Jesus' name I ask, believe, and receive them all. Amen.

More Encouragement: Exodus 15:2

Dig Deeper: Which of the Confidence in Action (CIA) pages resonates most with you? Be intentional—follow through on that particular CIA by taking action as your means of preparation and as a display of faith.

Confidence in Action

#7

Begin NOW to reduce expenses and to live off of one paycheck to help you determine how you will be able to stay at home to raise your child. Save the extra paychecks to cover "new baby expenses". If both of you need to work, start investigating safe and dependable child care by making unannounced visits to various facilities that are highly recommended by your personal friends/family/co-workers.

Reflections

A Victorious Mindset

"Fight the good fight of faith." ~ *1 Timothy 6:12* ~

Do you have the mindset of a fighter? Are you prepared to win at all costs? A great prizefighter prepares himself mentally as well as physically.

He wants to win. He does not let his opponent "get in his head." He does not listen to the lies and taunts of his opponent. How does he accomplish this? Just as he takes a lengthy amount of time to strengthen and train his body, he also takes the time to adjust his thoughts long before the fight. He tells himself things like "I'm a winner", "I will go the distance", and "I am stronger than my opponent." He has other people in his corner telling him those same things.

While you're in the battle against infertility, you too must adjust and renew your thinking. The Bible says in Romans 12:2, "And be not conformed to this world, but be transformed by the renewing of your mind..." You renew your mind by reading God's Word and meditating on it. This enables you to replace negative thoughts with positive thoughts that are based on God's promises. Do it as soon as you recognize that you're thinking negatively. Here's a good example:

> **Negative thought:** We have been trying to get pregnant for 2 years. I'm so ashamed! It hurts so

much to be around our friends who already have babies.

Immediately replace this thought with a positive one by speaking something from the Word of God...

Positive thought: God makes the barren woman to be a joyful mother of children *and that includes me.* (Psalm 113:9)

Renewing your mind with God's promises will enable you to block doubt and the fearful thoughts. Remember that God, who created and sustains the entire universe, is the One who loves you and blesses you. He will enable you to go the distance in this fight. Think about your past victories and answered prayers. Encourage yourself as David did (1 Samuel 30:6).

Speak God's Word about the situation knowing God has promised that as you speak it and believe it, His Word cannot be altered (Psalm 89:34). It will accomplish what He planned for you. Rest assured that His plans for you are good and will always give you hope for your future outcome (Jeremiah 29:11).

God never lies nor does He go back on His Word (Numbers 23:19), so use His Word to gain the prizefighter's edge—a victorious mindset!

Speak the Word: I fight the good fight of faith because I know my outcome through Jesus is always a victorious one.

More Encouragement: 2 Corinthians 2:14; Romans 8:37

Dig Deeper: Do you see yourself as a victim or victor?

Everyone But God Called Her Barren

"He settles the barren woman in her home as a happy mother of children. Praise the Lord!"
~ Psalm 113:9 (NIV) ~

Everyone, except God, must have called Elizabeth barren, repeatedly reminding her of the infertility of her womb. But God, the Creator of the universe and all that exists within it, did not agree with the label of "infertile" that Elizabeth's friends had put on her. He saw her from a different perspective.

Elizabeth endured being spurned and humiliated for many years. In her lifetime, women were expected to have babies at a young age. When that did not happen, a woman would have to suffer through being looked upon with reproach and being negatively classified as unfruitful and incapable of producing an heir for her husband. Producing an heir was of utmost importance in those times and great dishonor was placed upon a woman who could not produce.

But even though friends and family of Elizabeth may have looked down upon her, God saw the life-giving potential in her. He had a plan of honor for her...a son would be born to Elizabeth and her husband, Zechariah, and nothing would thwart God's plan (Luke 1:5-25). You may have experienced feeling ostracized or at least feeling like you know longer fit in with friends who now have children or are pregnant. But remember, God sees the life-giving potential in you just as He saw it in Elizabeth!

God has a plan and He is able *and willing* to transform your undesirable circumstances into blessings and reasons for praising Him.

Speak the Word: I praise God because He has made me a joyful mother of children.

More Encouragement: Ephesians 3:20

Dig Deeper: How do you feel about what God has said as it relates to *your* "life-giving potential"? What do you *say* about it?

Make the Exchange

"For he has rescued us from the kingdom of darkness and
transferred us into the Kingdom of his dear Son."
~ Colossians 1:13 (NLT) ~

Jesus has made the way for us to come out of the curse
of sin, sickness, poverty and death and to go into His
divine Blessing of righteousness, health, abundance,
and everlasting life. It's the Great Exchange.

Colossians 1:13 declares that we have been delivered from
the power of darkness and translated into Jesus' kingdom.
He has taken us from a life of darkness into a life of His
marvelous light!

If you are a believer in Christ, you chose to make this
exchange with God and allow Jesus to take your sin while
you received His right standing with God. Likewise, you
can choose to give Him this problem of infertility and allow
Him to deal with it on His own terms. God asks rhetorically
in Genesis 18:14, "Is any thing too hard for the Lord?" The
"thing" He was referring to was Sarah's infertility! The
problem of infertility is NOT too hard, too big, too
complex, or too long-lasting for God to eradicate. He's
lovingly and patiently waiting on you to trust Him and
completely turn it over to Him, to make the exchange so
that He can render infertility ineffective in your life.

How do you do that? Maybe part of my story will give you
some insight. First, I had to make the decision to cast the

problem of infertility onto Him. I then went to God in prayer to tell Him that I needed Him because I could no longer handle nor change the situation on my own (John 15:5). I had come to the end of my DIY efforts. I let my husband know that I had come to the end of self-effort and wanted to trust and rest in God about this situation. I also let God know that I was willingly and completely giving it over to Him, resting in the knowledge that He had the solution to infertility. I encourage you to trust Him to handle your situation.

Make the exchange and give Him:
> Your stress for His peace
> Your weakness for His strength
> Your sadness for His joy
> Your lack for His abundance
> Your confusion for His clarity
> Your loss for His victory

Speak the Word: The blood of Jesus has redeemed me. I have been transferred into His kingdom of Light. I live in the domain where God rules.

More Encouragement: 1 Peter 5:7; Psalm 55:22

Dig Deeper: What decisions do you need to make so that you make the exchanges as outlined above?

Pray *Now* on Behalf of Your Child

"And all thy children shall be taught of the LORD; and great shall be the peace of thy children." ~ Isaiah 54:13 ~

Recently, I pulled out my journal from the year that we had decided to start having children. In it, I found this entry for 6/2/86:

> *Parenting: 1 Samuel 1:27-28---"For this child I have prayed; and the Lord has given me my petition which I asked of Him. Therefore, I have lent him to the Lord; as long as he lives he shall be lent to the Lord."*

This passage of scripture is about Hannah who had asked God for a child and dedicated the child to God even *before* she became pregnant (1 Samuel 1:11). How can you dedicate or give something to someone else when you don't even have it in your hand? Hannah trusted God to honor her request and therefore she began to act on that trust. She acted by making a decision, *as she prayed her request,* that the child's life would be lived for God. Her expectation was that God would grant her request.

Mark 11:24 says that whatever things you desire, *when you pray, believe* that you receive them and you shall have them. Hannah believed as she prayed, she didn't have to wait to see it to believe it. That's called faith! She expected that God would come through for her and that her child would be a vessel for God to use. She prayed about the kind of person her child would become even before she became pregnant. Her prayers helped to determine not only the destiny of her son but also the destiny of the nation of Israel. The son that God blessed her to have was Samuel, who grew to become a mighty prophet of God. He was given the privilege to anoint David as king and later he became David's spiritual advisor.

Hannah declared the end from the beginning, just as God does. She is a good role model to have. You too can pray on behalf of your child even before you become pregnant. Find scriptures that relate to all the wonderful things you'd like to see in your child and pray them *out loud*. For example, do you want a child who loves God and is wise? Consider praying Proverbs 23:24-25: "The father of the righteous shall greatly rejoice and he that begets a wise child shall have joy in him."

Speak the Word: My child is righteous through faith in Jesus, set apart, without compromise and wise. I have great joy because of that child!

More Encouragement: 1 Samuel 1:1-28; Isaiah 44:3; 1 Thessalonians 3:12,13

Dig Deeper: What character traits would you like to pray for on behalf of your child even before you become pregnant?

Confidence in Action

#8

Pray that all of your children will choose
at a young age to accept Jesus.

Pray that all of your children will be
Spirit-filled and Spirit-led.

Reflections

_____

_____

_____

_____

_____

_____

_____

_____

_____

_____

_____

_____

_____

_____

_____

_____

_____

_____

_____

_____

Afterword: My Story

As a woman, I felt inadequate. I couldn't do the ONE thing that women can do that men can't—get pregnant. At times, I felt as if people pitied me, even though they did not. Sometimes I felt like an outcast, even though my friends welcomed me in their activities. But that was the painful part.

I had reached the age where all my friends had children so to attend any of their activities also meant being around their kids. I loved their children and had fun with them, but felt out of place not having a child of my own playing along with all the others. I remember trying to convince myself that it was OK—but it wasn't! It hurt!

There was never a firm diagnosis about why I was not getting pregnant. None of the tests produced conclusive results. I did have fibroids and as a result, had very heavy periods. There were also D&C surgeries and infections to live through. Going through the journey of infertility and all that comes along with it was not what I had signed up for in my perfect life.

But I decided that it was not going to be a source of depression nor a reason to become a hermit. I chose to enjoy life as it came and to do whatever it took to make the best of each day.

Doctor's reports were a source of frustration but God's report in the Bible was my source of hope. Choosing to stand on God's Word was an easy choice; actually *doing* it was not. It was a battle against my will, which wanted to do the easy thing and give up.

Making a stand for anything requires that you fight back against numerous attacks, not just one. I had to do just that—fight against numerous thoughts that were fearful, doubtful, and shame-filled *everyday*. Yes, I was ashamed that I could not get pregnant. No one else made me feel that way. It was self-inflicted.

Isn't it amazing what our own mind can do to inflict emotional pain on ourselves? The Word of God was my way out of that inner turmoil. I decided to keep "trying" no matter how long it took and watch God work it out.

I learned a lot during this struggle. The most important lesson learned was the power of speaking God's Word and believing His promises.

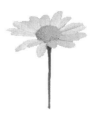

Finally Pregnant!

After five days of not having a period in November of 1987, I did a home pregnancy test and the test stick turned blue—its result was positive! I could hardly believe it. After all that time of "trying," after all the failed attempts and negative test results, I was finally pregnant! Once it actually happened, it did not seem real! But Freeman and I celebrated (very calmly). That day happened to be a Saturday and we were to play in a volleyball game with some church members. I chose to not play. I did not want to take any chances of falling or someone bumping into me.

After the game, I got a phone call from a close friend wondering what was going on since I didn't play. We told her the good news and swore her to secrecy. I couldn't allow myself to completely trust the test result until I could confirm it with a test at the doctor's office. I went in, having already told myself not to be too disappointed if it produced a negative result.

As I sat nervously in the examination room, the nurse came in and said with a big grin, "You're pregnant!" All the nurses in the office were so happy. They had seen me go through many pregnancy tests that turned out negative. Even my doctor was surprised that it finally happened! I was to meet Freeman for lunch that day and I could hardly wait to give him the good news. After we finished eating, I showed him the test results and congratulated him for officially being a daddy. He cried! It was a precious moment.

Just a week later, I experienced some spotting—small amounts of bleeding. Of course my first thought was, "Am I going to lose the baby?" Yes, even though I had experienced victory over infertility and had finally gotten pregnant, there was still fear of an attack from the devil on my body and now, also on my baby's life.

I had to choose whether to give in to the fear or trust God. I had to choose whether to accept the fearful thoughts, to cast them down, or just ignore them. I certainly did not want to give in and live with fearful thoughts. Ignoring them would have left them harboring in the recesses of my mind and having a place to silently grow into even larger, more fearful thoughts. I had to cast them down by re-directing my thoughts to God's love and power.

As the spotting continued during the next several weeks, I wrote in my journal that I had to remind myself of Colossians 2:15—"Jesus spoiled principalities and made a show of them openly". He did that for me *and* for my baby growing inside of me. I had to trust that this baby would make it through a full term pregnancy. It took much prayer by many people to boost our trust in God over the next few months as the spotting continued and even some cramping began. But God was faithful to His Word that Jesus had given us victory over infertility and childlessness! Our precious baby boy was born in June 1988, completely healthy and handsome.

To top it all off, God blessed us with another healthy and handsome son two years later. We were blessed with a healthy and beautiful daughter four years later. Those pregnancies occurred as soon as we started "trying" and both progressed smoothly. God can truly make a way when there seems to be no way!

Victory over infertility is indeed possible!

Appendix
Confessions of Faith

Speak some of these scriptures out loud each day. Affirm your belief that Jesus loves you and what God has said about your fertility is true and exists, even if you don't see it right now. Trust that if God said it, that's how He sees it in your life. Speak these scriptures in first person by inserting your name or, by saying I, my, me or mine, as appropriate.

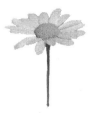

Isaiah 66:9—"Shall I bring to the time of birth, and not cause delivery?" says the LORD. "Shall I who cause delivery shut up the womb?" says your God."

Romans 4:19-21—"And not being weak in faith, he did not consider his own body, already dead (since he was about a hundred years old), and the deadness of Sarah's womb. He did not waver at the promise of God through unbelief, but was strengthened in faith, giving glory to God, and being fully convinced that what He had promised He was also able to perform."

Genesis 18:14—"Is any thing too hard for the LORD?"

Deuteronomy 7:13,14—"And He will love you and bless you and multiply you; He will also bless the fruit of your womb and the fruit of your land, your grain and your new wine and your oil, the increase of your cattle and the offspring of your flock, in the land of which He swore to your fathers to give you. You shall be blessed above all peoples; there shall not be a male or female barren among you or among your livestock."

Psalm 113:9—"He settles the barren woman in her home as a happy mother of children. Praise the LORD." [NIV]

Deuteronomy 7:15—"And the LORD will take away from you all sickness, and will afflict you with none of the terrible diseases of Egypt which you have known, but will lay them on all those who hate you."

Galatians 3:13—"But Christ has rescued us from the curse pronounced by the law. When he was hung on the cross, he took upon himself the curse for our wrongdoing. For it is written in the Scriptures, "Cursed is everyone who is hung on a tree." [NLT]

Mark 11:24—"Therefore I say to you, whatever things you ask when you pray, believe that you receive them, and you will have them."

Deuteronomy 28:2, 4—"All these blessings will come upon you and accompany you if you obey the LORD your God. [NIV] You will be blessed with many children and productive fields. You will be blessed with fertile herds and flocks." [NLT]

Leviticus 26:9—"For I will look on you favorably and make you fruitful, multiply you and confirm My covenant with you."

Psalm 139:13—"You made all the delicate, inner parts of my body and knit me together in my mother's womb." [NLT]

Genesis 30:22-23—"Then God remembered Rachel's plight and answered her prayers by giving her a child. She became pregnant and gave birth to a son. "God has removed my shame," she said." [NLT]

Luke 8:50—"But when Jesus heard it, He answered him, saying, "Do not be afraid; only believe, and she will be made well."

Psalm 107:20—"He sent his word, and healed them, and delivered them from their destructions."

Psalm 34:4—"I prayed to the LORD, and he answered me, freeing me from all my fears." [NLT]

Hebrews 11:11—"Because of faith also Sarah herself received physical power to conceive a child, even when she was long past the age for it, because she considered God who had given her the promise to be reliable and trustworthy and true to His word." [AMP]

Deuteronomy 28:11—"The LORD will grant you abundant prosperity—in the fruit of your womb, the young of your livestock and the crops of your ground—in the land he swore to your forefathers to give you." [NIV]

Luke 1:37—"For nothing is impossible with God." [NIV]

Luke 1:45—"You are blessed, because you believed that the Lord would do what he said." [NLT]

James 4:7—"Submit yourselves, then, to God. Resist the devil, and he will flee from you." [NIV]

2 Timothy 1:7—"For God has not given us a spirit of fear, but of power and of love and of a sound mind."

Psalm 103:2-5—"Praise the LORD, I tell myself, and never forget the good things he does for me. He forgives all my sins and heals all my diseases. He ransoms me from death and surrounds me with love and tender mercies. He fills my life with good things. My youth is renewed like the eagle's!" [NLT]

1 Peter 2:24—"who Himself bore our sins in His own body on the tree, that we, having died to sins, might live for righteousness—by whose stripes you were healed."

Proverbs 16:24—"Pleasant words are like a honeycomb, sweetness to the soul and health to the body." [RSV]

Proverbs 4:20-24—"My son, pay attention to what I say; listen closely to my words. Do not let them out of your sight, keep them within your heart; for they are life to those who find them and health to a man's whole body. Above all else, guard your heart, for it is the wellspring of life." [NIV]

Colossians 1:13—"He has delivered us from the dominion of darkness and transferred us to the kingdom of his beloved Son." [RSV]

John 17:17---"Sanctify them by Your truth. Your word is truth."

John 14:6—"Jesus told him, "I am the way, the truth, and the life. No one can come to the Father except through me." [NLT]

2 Corinthians 4:10—"Always carrying about in the body the dying of the Lord Jesus, that the life of Jesus also may be manifested in our body."

1 Corinthians 6:19—"Or don't you know that your body is the temple of the Holy Spirit, who lives in you and was given to you by God? You do not belong to yourself..."

Isaiah 50:7—"For the Lord GOD will help Me; Therefore I will not be disgraced; Therefore I have set My face like a flint, And I know that I will not be ashamed."

Jeremiah 30:17—"For I will restore health unto thee, and I will heal thee of thy wounds, saith the LORD."

Psalm 127:3—"Behold, children *are* a heritage from the LORD, the fruit of the womb *is* a reward."

Blessings to you and your children!

Thank you for reading

We invite you to share your thoughts and reactions

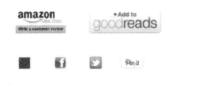

Continue to be encouraged!
Connect with Evangeline Colbert online:

Website:
http://www.EvangelineColbert.com

Bible Reading Plan on YouVersion:
http://bit.ly/1hK0jnO

Twitter:
http://twitter.com/evcolbert

Facebook:
http://facebook.com/hopefilledfocus

Find *A Seed of Hope* as an e-book at:

Amazon.com

Smashwords.com

Barnes and Noble.com

iTunes

Other books by Evangeline Colbert

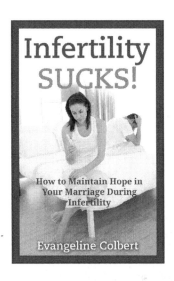

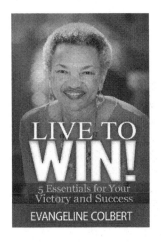